This is an excellent book: well-conceptualised, well-structured, well-researched, and well-written. In it, Rachel Cook brings her keen interest in and extensive knowledge of existential philosophy to bear on transactional analysis (TA); and, in doing so, fills some significant gaps in the espousal of existentialism by both Eric Berne and subsequent TA authors, including and centrally, by elaborating a model of adult development. As well as being theoretical, the book is deeply reflective, inviting the reader to think for – and about – themselves; and its accessibility and, therefore, practicality, is enhanced by the author's extensive use of case material drawn from her own practice, as well as poignant illustrations from her own life. In this Cook certainly achieves the – that is, her own – very human presence she sets out to do in the writing of book – and, now, in the reading of book. In this sense, I consider that the author demonstrates her humanism as well as her existentialism. In addition to her thorough and thoughtful discussion of adult development (comprising six chapters that form the second half of the book), there are other gems, including (in the first part of the book) chapters on authenticity, alienation, and encounter; on diagnosis, contracting, and treatment planning; and, a rare discussion (in TA), on self-disclosure. This is a book that warrants reading and re-reading, and is a must read for all TA practitioners, especially clinicians, as well as TA trainers and supervisors in all fields.

Keith Tudor, *PhD, TSTA(P), Professor of Psychotherapy, Auckland University of Technology, Auckland, Aotearoa New Zealand*

There is no doubt that Rachel Cook makes a real contribution to the TA literature with her ground-breaking existential approach – in particular she offers a model that charts the existential issues and challenges that accompany an adult's journey through the stages of life. She describes an in-depth methodology, from initial contact and contract, through to ending, 'for working with the existential dilemmas of adulthood, where growth can be about coming to terms with the existential givens of life rather than simply resolving psychodynamic disturbance' (p.82).

However, the book is more than that. It is a sort of rich autobiography that tracks the professional and personal development of the author as she develops a thoughtful and meaningful approach to psychotherapy, which will be useful not only for transactional analysts but any psychotherapist who wants to expand their approach to encompass existential thought. It is an enormously engaging read. Some parts are meticulously academic, such as Chapter 1, which plots the development of existential philosophy and psychotherapy within and outside of TA before embarking on her own ideas. Those parts are rich with theory and references; every concept is clearly explained and its history and evolution described; cultural differences are recognised and respected. Other parts are almost conversational – deeply personal and courageously self-disclosing, especially in the many vignettes and case studies that accompany and illustrate the ideas. It is a feast of a book.

Professor Charlotte Sills, *Hult Ashridge Business School, Metanoia Institute, UK*

Rachel Cook delivers a profound exploration of the existential dimension in psychotherapy, tracing its historical evolution from existential philosophy to therapeutic practice. She examines the development of Transactional Analysis (TA) from its existential foundations to a psychodynamic framework, skilfully reclaiming its potential as an existential psychotherapy. Tailored to different life stages—from adulthood transitions to maturation, self-clarification, and life's final phases—the book offers therapists a clear, actionable framework.

A core theme is what it means to approach therapy from an existential perspective, beginning with diagnosis and extending to treatment planning. The author integrates modern TA approaches, such as relational and co-creative therapy, creating a bridge between established principles and contemporary practices.

This work is a significant contribution to psychotherapy, embedding a proven theory into a comprehensive existential framework. It provides guidance for therapists navigating their own dilemmas and supporting clients in confronting existential challenges. By combining traditional and modern approaches, the book offers both theoretical depth and practical tools for today's practitioners.

Through insightful analysis and moving case studies, the author crafts an inspiring text that centres human existence in therapeutic work. It is a valuable resource for professionals seeking to deepen their understanding and enhance their practice.

Thorsten Geck, *TSTA (O), President of International Transactional Analysis Association, ITAA*

In this deeply personal and engaging book Rachel Cook offers us something we have been waiting for without knowing it. She returns to Eric Berne's existential thinking and locates TA, therapy and other professional encounters in a wider world than that of medical diagnosis or pathologising approaches. She takes us, step by step, through the grounding ideas of TA and explores a new perspective; key is her 'existential transactions' which cast a new light on therapy. Her focus, soundly rooted in existentialist philosophy, is on meaning, empathy and encounter as she asks 'how can we *not* be philosophical?' in what we do as practitioners and as ethical people. Building further on co-creative, relational and narrative approaches in TA, she inspires us as therapists and other practitioners to enter a 'more than human world' in our work through ongoing reflection and authentic contact with others.

Trudi Newton, *TSTA (E), Award-winning writer and educator in the field of Transactional Analysis, UK*

Existential Perspectives in Transactional Analysis

This book offers experienced practitioners and trainees in psychotherapy and counselling a new, deeply personal, and theoretically-grounded perspective on clinical work that integrates existential philosophy and psychotherapy into a relational transactional analysis.

The author employs a multidisciplinary perspective grounded in the traditions of Berne's transactional analysis, whilst providing an easily accessible explanation of existential psychotherapy and the existential givens of life. An innovative theory for the development of the adult self is offered that can be used to understand our human search for meaning and the existential life predicaments we all encounter as adults that may not originate from a difficult childhood. Using moving and personal clinical examples from her extensive professional experience as a psychotherapist, supervisor, and trainer, the author highlights the different therapeutic skills that can be used when working from this stance, making this a highly practical guide for all practitioners.

Whilst predominantly for psychotherapists, counsellors, and students on psychotherapy training courses, this will be essential reading for all practitioners working with human beings in groups, education, and organisations, as well as those who are new to the principles of existentialism and transactional analysis.

Rachel Cook is a Teaching and Supervising Transactional Analyst, UKCP registered Counsellor, Psychotherapist, Clinical Supervisor and Trainer. She has worked in psychotherapy and education for 30 years and facilitates training courses in the New Forest, UK.

Innovations in Transactional Analysis: Theory and Practice
Series Editor: William F. Cornell

This book series is founded on the principle of the importance of open discussion, debate, critique, experimentation, and the integration of other models in fostering innovation in all the arenas of transactional analytic theory and practice: psychotherapy, counseling, education, organizational development, health care, and coaching. It will be a home for the work of established authors and new voices.

Revitalization Through Transactional Analysis Group Treatment: Human Nature and Its Deterioration
Giorgio Piccinino

Working with Dreams in Transactional Analysis: From Theory to Practice for Individuals and Groups
Anna Emanuela Tangolo and Francesca Vignozzi

Conceptualizing Ego States in Transactional Analysis: Three Systems in Interaction
José Grégoire

A Transactional Analysis of Motherhood and Disturbances in the Maternal
Emma Haynes

A Living History of Transactional Analysis Psychotherapy: Engaging Reflectively with Theory and Methodology
Steff Oates and Diana Deaconu

Existential Perspectives in Transactional Analysis: The Development of the Adult Self and the Human Search for Meaning
Rachel Cook

https://www.routledge.com/Innovations-in-Transactional-Analysis-Theory-and-Practice/book-series/INNTA

Existential Perspectives in Transactional Analysis

The Development of the Adult Self and the Human Search for Meaning

Rachel Cook

Routledge
Taylor & Francis Group

LONDON AND NEW YORK

Designed cover image: With thanks to J. O'Connor for permission to use her painting, 'Tilly', September 2024

First published 2026
by Routledge
4 Park Square, Milton Park, Abingdon, Oxon, OX14 4RN

and by Routledge
605 Third Avenue, New York, NY 10158

Routledge is an imprint of the Taylor & Francis Group, an informa business

© 2026 Rachel Cook

British Library Cataloguing-in-Publication Data
A catalogue record for this book is available from the British Library

ISBN: 978-1-032-75692-9 (hbk)
ISBN: 978-1-032-75691-2 (pbk)
ISBN: 978-1-003-47521-7 (ebk)

DOI: 10.4324/9781003475217

Typeset in Times New Roman
by SPi Technologies India Pvt Ltd (Straive)

To Billy and Ben
For your past, present, and future

Contents

Acknowledgements

Thank you to my parents. For gifting me with life, love, curiosity, intellect, and spirituality, and for teaching me how to laugh through the ups and downs of existence. I am so lucky to have had the security of your supportive and challenging loving presence for so many years. Thank you for demonstrating how to embrace with vitality every stage of life. You are an inspiration.

Thank you to my siblings. The only others who have been a constant throughout every stage of my life. I am so grateful to you and your spouses for being variously role models, advisors, sounding boards, critical friends, fierce competitors, comforters, loyal companions, and playmates. Life is so much more fun and manageable with my big brother and sisters alongside me.

Thank you to my sons. Parenting you has been the most joyful, rewarding, and challenging privilege of my life. Thank you for your creative vibrancy, intelligent humour, enquiring minds, and honest confrontation that keeps me on my toes, pushes me to better myself, and helps me see the world and relationships in a different way. Your encouragement with my work and writing has been profoundly touching and has kept me going through the hard times.

Thank you to my therapist and supervisors. You have been my faithful accompaniers, cheerleaders, thought-provoking challengers, educators, and helpmates through the twists and turns of my life and work. Laurence Hegan, Sally Dhruev, and Suzanne Boyd, your humanity and genuine care has taught me about authentic encounter, empowerment, creativity, and commitment. Charlotte Sills, I would not have pursued this book if it had not been for your mentoring, encouragement, and inspiration.

Thank you to my supervisees. Our relationships have been a joy and a challenge, and have deeply enriched my life. You have made me think, cry, and laugh, and learning from and with you has made me a better teacher, supervisor, therapist, writer, and person. Thank you particularly to those who have contributed to this book: Laurence Taylor, Katie Angus, Sarita Markouizos, Lucy Cassels, Deniz Sarper, Ellie Pendred, Holly Underwood, Chris Bancroft, Sarah Willey, Charlie Allen, Katie Daley, Alice Joyce, Ali Strong, Caz Bowden, and Katherine Staples. I have been so touched by your encouragement in sharing my excitement and struggles of writing. Your ongoing trust in me and your commitment through the difficulties of relating has been deeply impactful.

Thank you to my clients. Without your courage, honesty, vulnerability, generosity, inspiration, challenge, and motivation there could be no book. In trusting me to accompany you in your search for meaning, you have gifted me with immeasurable meaning in my life.

Thank you to my students. You constantly make me realise how much there is to learn in life and how little I know, and I am so grateful that you never stop pushing me to keep developing.

Thank you to my editor, Bill Cornell. Your inspiring writing, editing, and humanity has enabled me to become an author. Thank you for having the belief in me, and for sharing yourself with me in a way that unlocked my creativity. Your honesty, encouragement, thoughtful questioning, and commitment to live through the dark as well as the light has helped me better understand the realities, uncertainties and limits of life, psychotherapy, and writing.

Thank you to my friends and colleagues. Annie Jenkinson, Kathryn Walters, Keith Tudor, Emma Haynes, Jane Skinner, Jenny Cole, and Nicola Grainger, you have been immensely encouraging and supportive with my writing, and inspiring in my life and work. It is a wonderful gift to have people you can call on when the going gets tough, and I appreciate you all enormously. Richard, you have been poignantly present with me throughout the writing of this book.

Thank you to my feline companions. To Stan, my most faithful furry friend, who sits with me and on me while I write, and has enriched my life through his embodied presence on every stage of my journey as a psychotherapist and author. To Charlie, who makes me laugh every day and teaches me what it is to enjoy life. And to Tilly, who in her life and death, helped me understand more deeply the meaning of relatedness and transcendence.

Introduction
Death, life, and companionship

Companionship in death and life

My beloved cat, Tilly, was recently killed by a car outside my home. Her sudden and brutal death brought the pain and joy of existence into sharper focus, as it does for anyone contending with the loss of a cherished person or animal companion – or indeed any unwanted or challenging life event. We are presented simultaneously with the pain of the present loss, the precious memories of the past, and the anxieties of the future. We are reminded that our own and our loved ones' existence in this world is finite, and we are faced with the disturbing reality of the uncertainty and unpredictability of life at the same time as the inevitability of change. We may feel the urgency of making the most of our limited existence, but feel an anxious responsibility for the decisions that determine the outcome of our life, and struggle to find meaning in a world where death is the only certainty. This can make us feel isolated and alone. Yet there is also a universality about these existential dilemmas, as every human being will face them throughout the different stages of their life – even though some may find ingenious ways to distract from, avoid, or deny these tensions. Relationship can soothe the pain of existential isolation, and the human companionship of therapy and consultation can be one way to help those in existential distress. Seeing that we share the same predicaments and tensions, and that we have survived, grown, and found meaning through the struggles of humanity, can help people discover their own meaning in a more vital and authentic existence. I have attempted to bring such a human presence in the writing of this book. My hope is that, in sharing some of my own struggles and those of the people whom I have accompanied, you, the reader, will feel less alone in facing courageously your own existential life challenges. And as you do so, I hope that you as therapist will feel better equipped to offer your authentic humanity to your clients as they encounter theirs. For in our inevitable and universal struggles with being human we have more that unites us than divides. We *all* need companions alongside us to help us navigate the rugged and diverse terrains of human existence.

DOI: 10.4324/9781003475217-1

Sometimes our companions along the way are other living beings. Tilly had been such a companion for me. For 12 years she was a silent witness to my life, accompanying me through the delights, despair, and challenges of my transition from early adulthood into mid-life: divorce, bereavement, single parenting, new jobs, menopause, health scares, my eldest child leaving home, my mother's decline through dementia, becoming a great-aunt seven times over, and transitioning from psychotherapist into supervisor, teacher, and writer. Her companionship has helped me to live a more abundant existence. She brought joy, fun, and playfulness into my fractured family after the ending of my marriage, and offered comfort and healing amidst the grief. Her beauty, velvety soft fur, soothing purr, and endearing squeaky miaows provided aesthetic and sensory pleasure. Our shared enjoyment of her helped my sons and I connect with each other throughout their childhood, adolescence, and emerging adulthood. In enjoying being with us, she helped us feel loved, and in needing our care she gave us all opportunities to love, protect, and nurture. She offered me a sense of solidarity in having another embodied female presence in the house, alleviated loneliness, and inspired creativity in sitting alongside me as I wrote this book. She embodied and invited curiosity, exploring her world with passion, freedom, fear, and pleasure. And she taught me about relatedness. I learnt to appreciate her gentle presence alongside me rather than trying to insist on her being on my lap. And in her regular gifting of dead rodents – not the most thoughtful gift for someone with a phobia of dead animals! – I learnt to tolerate better that we all have a shadow side, and that life and death are inextricably intertwined. Nowhere was this more apparent than in the trauma of her death, when the love, support, and kindness of neighbours, friends and strangers in my time of vulnerability helped me grow through the loss, grief, and destruction. In the ending of her life, Tilly gifted me with a final beautiful spiritual encounter. Through her death, life, and companionship, I felt the expansive wonder of human existence: playfulness, creativity, relatedness, emotionality, thoughtfulness, sensuality, vulnerability, and spirituality. It is the reason I have chosen her picture for the cover of this book, a moving gift painted for me by a much-loved client on the occasion of Tilly's death.

The thirst of the soul

It is an immense privilege of our profession to be a human companion for others. But to accompany another in an exploration of their own existential dilemmas, life tensions, and search for meaning and growth we need more than a psychodynamic approach to psychotherapy. We need a curiosity and wonder at life, death, and human existence that is at the heart of philosophical thinking. My hope is that this book inspires and provokes this spirit of inquiry. Philosophy is for everyone: it is a childlike search for truth and a love of wisdom. I cannot see how anyone can be a psychotherapist without this curiosity. Such a thirst of the soul drives my work and life and has been with me as long as I can remember. A considerable part of my childhood and adolescence was spent wondering about the big questions of existence, leading to various spiritual and religious explorations, and culminating in more formal studies of philosophy at university. My love of learning and personal development led me into the teaching profession, where, over many years, I experimented with teaching history, politics, and mathematics, before realising that relationship, mentoring, and pastoral care were the aspects of my work that gave me most meaning. I also found this meaning in parenting. My spontaneous response to my deep-thinking son's philosophical questions about the meaning of life was always "relationship": relationship with humans, relationship with animals, relationship with nature, and relationship with the spiritual. And it was the sad breakdown of a relationship that led me unintentionally into transactional analysis (TA) and the world of psychotherapy. Relationship therapy with my then husband in our early thirties did not ultimately save our marriage, but it gave me life in a way that I could never have imagined. Our therapist happened to be a transactional analyst and I hungrily devoured the theory and reading she offered. The wonderful simplicity yet complexity of TA theory made sense to me, helped me understand myself and my ways of relating, and opened my eyes to previously unconsidered and unconscious intrapsychic and interpersonal relational dynamics. Thirsty for more, I enrolled on a Master's degree in TA psychotherapy, and so began a change in career that transformed my personal and professional life in the most stimulating, challenging, and enriching ways. I could not have imagined as a young adult the meaning I would find in middle age in teaching, supervising, mentoring, and accompanying others in *their* search for meaning.

The existential limitations of transactional analysis

As much as TA has been transformational for me and for those who have shared their life and work with me, at times I have searched for more. When my marriage eventually ended and I faced my own existential and spiritual crisis, the theories, methodologies, and methods of TA were not enough for me. I could not find in the literature the comfort, challenge, and wisdom that I needed to help me make sense of the realities of my present experiences of death, life, destruction, and creativity. At the same time, I was increasingly finding that clients were coming to therapy for help with existential life issues that were not necessarily or solely linked to psychodynamic issues emanating from childhood. They were struggling with the issues of existence – death, illness, pandemics, wars, financial crises, responsibility, political corruption, immorality, climate change, artificial intelligence, isolation, alienation. They were facing the very real and often universal challenges of adulthood as they transitioned through different life stages and came up against the accompanying choices, responsibilities, tensions, and struggles with relatedness and meaning-making. When facing these existential life crises and dilemmas, I realised that what I and many of my clients needed was not simply to dig around in our past in an attempt to find links with the present, but to be accompanied in our spiritual and existential quest by someone who could help us examine with courage and tenacity the tensions, challenges, tasks, and dilemmas of present life. Yet, despite TA being founded with promising existential philosophical roots, it did not currently offer me the thinking, philosophy, or methods to help me to do this. Eric Berne, the psychoanalyst and psychiatrist who founded TA in the US in the 1950s and 1960s, had proposed that TA was an existential psychotherapy and encouraged trainees to familiarise themselves with it, yet his writing drove TA down the route of cognitive-behavioural and psychody-namic psychology rather than existential philosophy. His contemporaries and later TA authors furthered his theories on the psychological development of the child, but I could not find in TA any thinking on the developmental stages of adulthood. Instead, I turned to the teachings of existential psychotherapy and adult developmental psychology to help me in my own existential striv-ings. In doing so, I discovered that I was more able to help my clients who were grappling with their own existential crises and challenges of different adult life stages. This book is the culmination of the last 20 years of my soul-searching, explorations, experimentations, and personal and professional relationships.

The companionship of therapy: an existential provocation

In this book, I offer an existential and adult developmental perspective to TA. My aim is not to replace a psychodynamic approach to TA – far from it – but to provoke a wider and deeper inquiry into the multiple possibilities for a cli-ent's difficulties. I want to inspire both psychodynamic and existential thera-pists and consultants to creatively tailor their stance to the unique needs of each individual, whether that is psychodynamic, existential, or an adult devel-opmental life stage approach – or more often than not, a combination of all three. I provide personal and clinical examples to help us consider that beyond the possible psychodynamic and historical reasons for our clients' difficulties or distress, there may alternatively or additionally be challenges emanating from their particular adult life stage or the universal dilemmas of being human. Likewise, it is important to remember that underneath what at first seems to be existential angst may also be psychodynamic disturbance. We need to consider both/and, not either/or. This was illustrated for me by Tilly's death, where I experienced a multi-faceted grief. Existentially, I was grieving the present loss of my feline companion, and coming to terms with the reality of death and the unexpectedness of sudden trauma. Life felt dangerous and precarious. Psychodynamically, I also uncovered an unprocessed childhood grief for my first cat who died in similar traumatic circumstances when I was six years old, leaving me with confusion and unfinished business around death and separa-tion. For the first time, Tilly's death enabled me to make sense of how previous unsupported losses and separations linked to my subsequent lifelong phobia of dead animals, and how it sedimented an already-present separation anxiety that accompanied me into adulthood. And existentially, this circled back into a growing awareness that underneath these anxieties was an ever-present fear of my own death, the ultimate separation. Perhaps it would be reasonable to surmise that such unfinished business and existential angst may have led to my choices to study philosophy at university, become a psychotherapist, and write a psychotherapy book about existentialism! If so, I am grateful that they did. For they have helped me to make meaning and face with greater equanimity the reality of death and the limitations of life. And this has enabled me to live life more passionately and plentifully.

My hope is that my thoughts, stories, and existential provocations in the forthcoming chapters will enable you and your clients to do the same. As psychotherapists and consultants, we are gifted the privilege of accompanying people on part of their life's journey, not as a guide that shows them *our* way, but as a companion that offers the support and confrontation of our embodied presence to help them find theirs. Our presence offers the possibility of a different relational experience from the past, and in offering our humanity, we hold up a confronting mirror to invite people to explore their own human questions and challenges, their strengths and frailties. We need to have the humility to acknowledge that it is our fallible humanity that is the best thing that we offer, not our theories, techniques, interventions, or interpretations. When Tilly died, the most transformational experience for me came from the humanity of neighbours, friends, and strangers who enveloped me with care and kindness. I was not alone with death as I had been as a six year old. These fellow human beings – all of whom had experienced their own significant bereavements – carried her lifeless body off the road, wrapped her in a beautiful silver silk cloth, held me as they broke the news of her death, made me cups of tea, talked about her life, dug her grave, and stood alongside me as we buried my beloved companion in my garden. They were able to help me face death because they had touched it themselves in an even more profound way – and they knew the power of companionship in helping people to do so.

If we are to accompany people in a similar way in our therapy and consultation rooms, we need to have examined our own existential challenges and dilemmas, and acknowledge and accept more fully the possibilities and limitations of past, present, and future. We need to be on the road to acceptance that death is a certainty and time is limited for all of us, thus enabling us to choose to live the time we have left with greater vigour, freedom, responsibility, authenticity, and personal meaning. If we cannot face death and life's limitations, how can we help our clients with their own living? As I wrote this introduction, I had a dream that I was back at school, important exams were approaching, and I had not revised. A typical anxiety dream for me. Yet my dream took a novel turn when I calmly decided that exams were not the most important thing in life and chose instead to spend my limited time having an exhilarating walk at the beach. Anxiety emerged in the dream once again when I returned from my walk to what I thought was a parking ticket on my car. Yet my anxiety turned to joy when, on closer inspection, it transpired to be a gift rather than a penalty: a loving note from my sister accompanied by a bunch of daffodils, my favourite spring flowers. An existential perspective to dreams sees them as important as our waking life, and this dream for me symbolises quite beautifully the anxiety we can feel about our responsibility for our life choices. We are free to choose our direction, yet we can never know what the outcome of our decision will be. We are thus always faced with the possibility of regrets for the choices we make in life, which can lead to paralysis and stagnation. I had such an existential predicament in choosing to write this book. To devote the time necessary, I have had to sacrifice other opportunities which I will now never get to experience or accomplish. I will never know for sure whether I made the right choice; perhaps I will eventually feel existential guilt that I have not made the best use of my limited time, or spent more time with the people I love. There have certainly been moments when making myself write has felt like turgid exam revision, but mostly the experience has been more like the enlivening and exhilarating beach walk. Yet would my other options have been even more vitalising? I will never know. There is also still anxiety about how it will be received by its readers: parking ticket or daffodils? No doubt one as well as the other, for it is a certainty that life provides us with both. It is such existential dilemmas, tensions, and impasses that are woven throughout the fabric of this book.

The developmental stages of the book

Quite fittingly, writing this book has felt like giving life to something, and I have seen the evolution of its chapters and my ideas and creativity in much the same way that I see the development of a person throughout their lifespan. It has been both a linear and circular process, recycling old ideas and experiences in the creation of something new. And always aiming towards its final ending. The end result is a book of thirteen chapters in three sections.

Section 1 An introduction to existential psychotherapy and transactional analysis

The first five chapters offer an outline of the thinking, theories, and methods of existential psychotherapy, and the similarities and differences with TA. My aim has been to make this accessible to those with no knowledge of existential psychotherapy, for people new to TA, and to anyone for whom both approaches are novel. At its core, existential philosophy is for everyone, because it is about the universal issues of human experience. Likewise, the philosophy of TA is about accessibility and mutuality, and I hope practitioners from any modality may benefit from the summaries and ideas that I offer.

Section 2 The development of the adult

The second section of the book, Chapters 6 to 11, introduce the thinking and research of adult developmental psychology into both TA and an existential approach. Using clinical and personal examples from my own life and relational experiences, I delve deeper into the potential joys, tensions, and challenges of each of the five adult life stages, and the various existential dilemmas, challenges, and tensions that we may encounter at any stage of life. I do not suggest a life plan with rigid phases, but offer possibilities and ideas for us to consider as we navigate the different terrains of our own individual life journey, and assist our clients in traversing theirs. Whilst each odyssey is unique, my hope is that practitioners – and ultimately their clients – will find a sense of connection and shared humanity through my offering of sometimes deeply personal illustrations.

Section 3 Death and life

The final section, Chapters 12 and 13, is appropriately focused on life and death: the fundamental, inter-related and inextricably entwined aspects of existence. I had planned to write first about the erotic life force, then end the book with the chapter on death – the final ending for us all. As I wrote, however, it seemed more fitting to end with life. Facing into the ending of death can help us discover our erotic life force that enables us to live the time we have left with greater vitality and creativity. This is my hope for you and your clients.

My wish is that in reading this book you experience a fellow human who offers you companionship in the face of life and death and in the inevitable existential struggles that we all encounter. I hope that my writing enables you to make greater sense of your own life and its inevitable freedoms and limitations so that you can bring the fullness of your humanity into your relationships with your clients. In doing so, I hope you and they will be able to discover greater passion and creativity for life; increased resilience and resourcefulness to tolerate the seemingly intolerable; and a growing capacity for intimate, authentic connection with yourselves, other people, animals, nature, the arts, our wonderfully diverse world, and the mysteries of the spiritual realm that is beyond our human existence. Above all, I hope you find meaning in the work that you do. For surely there is no greater creative and spiritual meaning in life than being a companion for others as they navigate their individual journey through life towards the inevitable death that will one day come to us all.

Section 1

An introduction to existential psychotherapy and transactional analysis

Chapter 1

What is existentialism and existential psychotherapy?

What is philosophy?

I think I have been a philosopher since the age of five. I distinctly remember walking down my road on my own (that's what we did in the 1970s!) thinking 'who am I?'. I was enthralled and curious at the idea that I had a body that was walking but was also aware of a "me" that was far bigger and more mysterious, that enabled me to think and consider myself. I was becoming conscious of my consciousness. Studying philosophy at university 13 years later, I realised Descartes (1637) had beaten me to it by about 300 years with his philosophical ideas "Cogito, ergo sum": "I think therefore I am"!

Philosophy is for everyone, even (or especially) five year olds. If only we could retain the curiosity, awe, and wonder at the world of a five year old. Instead, many fear philosophy as being too difficult to grasp, too academic or intellectual, with too many big words ending in 'ology', little relevance to everyday life, or too negative, depressing or anxiety-provoking. As one of my supervisees exclaimed when I suggested she explore an existential perspective with her client: "Oh no, that's not for me, philosophy is far too vague and lofty". You may be able to imagine the friendly yet confrontational response I offered!

Far from being "lofty", I consider the philosophical attitude to have great depth and profundity as it is about questioning extensively life, ourselves, others, the world around us, and what may be beyond. It is about not taking things at face value but digging deeper to achieve greater awareness and understanding. The word philosophy comes from the Greek for a "love of wisdom": intimately and dynamically exploring the big questions of life in a search for truth, or an attempt to understand the socially and culturally constructed truth (Foucault, 1972). Who am I? Who am I in relationship with other people and the world? What does it mean to be a human being for my finite time on earth? What is the meaning of life? Do I have free will or is my life determined by a higher power or other causes? What is right and wrong? What is truth? What do I believe happens after death? Does God or a Higher Power exist? How can I best live a life of meaning, value, and purpose?

DOI: 10.4324/9781003475217-3

I believe that the most important quality of an effective therapist or consultant is the capacity for reflective thinking and reflexivity. Philosophy enables us to reflect on life and our guiding principles, beliefs, and values, bringing the unthought into consciousness. Through philosophical thinking we can gain greater understanding of the historically and culturally constructed knowledge and value systems we live by, gaining wisdom and knowledge about our human existence and how we relate to the world and other people. Without philosophical thinking we would not have the boundaries of our profession; our ethical codes originate from the branch of philosophy called "ethics". Ethical philosophical thinking ensures we can consider the moral principles that guide our professional behaviour, how our role is differentiated from friendship, romance, or collegial relationship, and how we think about "right and wrong". It is also because of philosophical thinking and principles that we can know why we do what we do as practitioners, why we hold the views and attitudes we do, and how we think about our political stance and relationship with power. It is in finding the answers to these questions that we can become congruent and ethical practitioners; so how can we *not* be philosophical?

Philosophical principles and assumptions of transactional analysis (TA)

Philosophy is the foundation of any psychotherapeutic modality, educational methodology, or organisation. Rogers (1959) argued that we cannot engage in psychotherapy without giving operational evidence of an underlying value orientation and view of human nature, and that such views should be open and explicit, rather than covert and implicit. Unfortunately, training often leaves out the philosophical to favour the psychological, behavioural, biological, social, political, intellectual, or spiritual causes for distress (van Deurzen & Adams, 2016). TA, in particular, has traditionally focused on the intrapsychic, interpersonal, and intersubjective at the expense of considering the human condition and its wider philosophical and socio-political context. We need both/and, not either/or. However, Eric Berne based his philosophy of TA on the thinking of some of the great philosophers, particularly Søren Kierkegaard: people are OK; everyone has the capacity to think; and early decisions can be changed. He also outlined philosophical principles of mutuality, the client being an active participant, and open communication. To become a Certified Transactional Analyst (CTA), trainees are required to describe and critique their own personal style of TA in relation to these philosophical assumptions and principles, while Teaching and Supervising Transactional Analysts (TSTA) must be able to explain their philosophy of supervision and training. What is being looked for is a practitioner who is congruent, coherent, and consistent, with integration between their personal philosophy of life and practice, their professional methodology, practical application, and adopted theories (Tudor, 2010, p. 275). At the centre of it all is our personal, unique self: our 'Being'

(Heidegger, 1927/2010). In short, are we the same person inside and outside the therapy, supervision, and training room? Are we being authentic to our personhood, beliefs, and values?

Our personal philosophy of life

Before we can know our philosophy of therapy, teaching, consultation, or supervision, we need to be able to wonder about our personal philosophy of life. I ask my trainees (and clients) to consider their three core values in life: what are the things that drive you, create passion, give you energy? What are the principles that drive you to distraction or make you feel angry, stifled, or unseen when others do not demonstrate them? What would you want people to write about you in your obituary? One of my clients once said to me after a particularly hard-hitting confrontation: "On your grave stone it will say, 'Loving and kind but doesn't fuck around!'" We belly laughed together, and she also made me think: would I be content if that is what I am remembered for? I think so, as my core values are authenticity, integrity, honesty, and love (and because I also have a slight rebellious streak, I have chosen four, not three!).

The foundational value for me is authenticity, emanating from some of my childhood experiences of living with the tension and anxiety from ulterior communication, as well as explosions of conflict followed by withdrawal. Amidst this, my older brother was honest and authentic with me, sometimes brutally so, but there was no room for misunderstanding that at times he found me an irritating little sister! Despite it being difficult sometimes, I appreciated the openness and knowing where I stood. Today, open communication and "realness" help alleviate my anxiety and enables me to be more spontaneous and freer to be my authentic self. No wonder I was drawn to the open communication of TA, to a two-person way of working (Stark, 2000) and to the authenticity of the existential approach (the focus of Chapter 2).

What are the main words you find yourself using repeatedly? I sometimes offer trainees words to help them see which jump out at them, such as the TA's ethical principles and values (European Association of Transactional Analysis, 2007/2011; International Transactional Analysis Association, 2014): respect, empowerment, protection, responsibility, commitment in relationship, and dignity, health, security, self-determination, and mutuality. Other values people have chosen include love, creativity, fun, integrity, commitment, reliability, vulnerability, autonomy, authenticity, honesty, loyalty, kindness, courage, spirituality, compassion, accountability, wisdom, assertiveness, trust, self-discipline, generosity, gratitude, sustainability, wealth, humility, success, safety, altruism, patience, determination, freedom, power, fairness, justice, uniqueness, inclusivity.

Once chosen, it is important to reflect on why your history and life script make these values so key to you. How are they linked, and how were they demonstrated (or not demonstrated) in your early and later life? How do these values impact the way you live now: the activities you are involved in, the relationships you sustain or leave, the work you do, and your personal style of psychotherapy, consultation, supervision, or training? What may be the ways that you are not currently living by your values? What is the shadow side of these values (because there inevitably will be!)? My philosophical values help inspire my clients, supervisees, and trainees to be courageous in being real with me and others, thereby helping them and their clients become more authentic, more fully human, and with greater integrity. My client said she liked that I "don't fuck around" because my honesty challenged her, and, alongside my love, it helped her to trust me and feel safe because she knew where she stood. The shadow side is that my authenticity and honesty can sometimes be too much for people, or my integrity can mean my standards can be too high. One of my supervisees used the powerful illustration of an old-fashioned horse race at the amusement arcade, where one horse shoots off ahead, leaving the others struggling to catch up. When I shoot off ahead in my clamouring for authenticity, I can be experienced as too direct, challenging, or intimidating, leaving the other feeling inadequate or myself being dehumanised through projections (good and bad) – the very opposite of my intention. We can get too stuck and rigid on one extreme of our philosophical values and need to integrate other values to counter this: for me, this is compassion and vulnerability. The "loving kindness" as well as the "doesn't fuck around"! Luckily, I have an array of authentic trainees, supervisees, and children who remind me when I need more balance!

Once in awareness, we can decide which of our philosophical values we want to keep, which we want to discard or integrate, and which we want to loosen. Most often, the values do not change, it is simply the awareness around them that is heightened, and sometimes the ferocity of chasing these values at all costs can be softened. Having greater awareness of our philosophy of life can help us understand our philosophy of therapy, supervision or teaching; as the saying goes: if we are going to spend our life climbing a ladder, we need to make sure we are leaning it against the right wall.

Our core values do not fully describe our essence as a human being, however. We are far more than the sum of our values or qualities and we cannot be reduced to a list of attributes. The German philosopher, Martin Heidegger, and the French philosopher, Jean-Paul Sartre, proposed that "existence comes before essence" (van Deurzen & Adams, 2016, p. 10): the *essence* of our being and our values (our identity) comes through our *existence* in relationship with others and the world. Heidegger (1927/2010) referred to this as our 'Being', our 'Being-in-the-World', and our 'Being-in-the-World-with-Others'. It is the exploration of the nature of this existence as a human being in a world with other human beings (the "human condition") that is the basis of the branch of philosophy called "existentialism".

A brief history of existentialism

Thinking, discussing, and writing about the big questions of life helped develop existential philosophical thinking into a philosophical movement in the 20th century. The great minds of philosophers such as Søren Kierkegaard, Friedrich Nietzsche, Karl Jaspers, Martin Heidegger, Gabriel Marcel, Jean-Paul Sartre, and Simone de Beauvoir delved into questions around existence, meaning and significance, human relating, death, free will and determinism, right and wrong, truth, God, and uniqueness. The ideas and answers they came up with were beautifully diverse and often contradictory, just like human beings themselves. Some (like Kierkegaard, Buber, and Marcel) were deeply religious, others (like Sartre, Nietzsche, and Camus) were committed atheists. Some emphasised the need for individuality (Kierkegaard and Nietzsche), others for relationship (Buber, Marcel, and Jaspers). Some consider existence to be ultimately meaningless (Sartre and Camus), others (like Marcel) place great emphasis on hope (Cooper, 2017, p. 13).

One of the criticisms sometimes levied at existential ideas is that they are too pessimistic. Certainly, if you simply read Schopenhauer's views that existence has no value you might be forgiven for drawing that conclusion! My view, however, is that most existential thought is about hope in humanity. Whilst there is an acceptance of the inevitable suffering, struggles, aloneness, and tensions of life, there is also the encouragement that accepting these difficulties, and the inevitability of our death, can help us live more fully, vitally, and authentically, which is empowering and deeply fulfilling. I encourage you to hold this hope in mind as I go on to offer a brief summary of the significant existential philosophers and their main philosophical ideas.

Kierkegaard and Nietzsche

The founders of existential philosophy in the 19th century are widely agreed to be the Danish philosopher, Søren Kierkegaard (1813–1855), and the German philosopher, Friedrich Nietzsche (1844–1900). Both were individualistic, acknowledging our individual free will and our own responsibility for making life meaningful (rather than following the "crowd" for Kierkegaard (1844/1980), or the "herd mentality" for Nietzsche (1886/1989)). Nietzsche argued that as "God is dead", morality is a human construct and life is essentially meaningless (nihilism), it is up to individuals to think for themselves and make choices as to how to live their lives according to their own values and beliefs. Kierkegaard acknowledged the inevitable fear, anxiety, or 'angst' that the responsibility of this freedom could evoke, believing we can learn from it if we can better tolerate it and if we can find our own personal sense of and relationship to God. Whilst Nietzsche was firmly atheist, he later said that suffering makes us stronger and that art was the one thing that could relieve our suffering.

Husserl

The Austrian–German logician and mathematician, Edmund Husserl (1859–1938), developed "phenomenology". Husserl's (1931/2012) process of phenomenological inquiry is about description rather than interpretation, where we aim to suspend or "bracket" our own judgement, biases or preconceived notions to really hear and understand the individual's subjective world and their lived experience with an open mind (Spinelli, 2015). Husserl first coined the term "intersubjectivity" for the process of shared understanding of thoughts and feelings between two "subjects" (facilitated by empathy). He suggested that this makes possible the objectivity of being in the Other's position and the understanding of consciousness itself, the only thing of which we can be certain.

Heidegger

Husserl's assistant, the German philosopher, Martin Heidegger (1889–1976), argued that consciousness can never be separated from its context as we are always involved with the world and others (our "Being-in-the-World", Heidegger, 1927/2010). His belief in unconscious experience influenced psychoanalysis as well as existentialism, and his concepts of "Dasein" (or "Being there") and "thrownness" influenced the Swiss psychiatrists, Ludwig Binswanger and Medard Boss, in the creation of the first existential psychotherapy, Daseinsanalysis (described later). Heidegger suggested that humans are inevitably and unavoidably thrown into a world where we have to cope with the struggles of life, relationships and our "Being-toward-Death" (a state called "facticity"). Similar to Kierkegaard and Nietzsche, he was an advocate for authenticity in individuality, believing that living our lives like the masses was "inauthenticity" or "fallenness", and to live an authentic life meant truly engaging with the anxiety surrounding our awareness of time and our inevitable death.

Buber

Existential thinking became decidedly more relational thanks to the Austrian Jewish philosopher and theologian, Martin Buber (1878–1965). He emphasised the relational nature of human existence, describing the intersubjective space between two people (or the "between") as greater than the contribution of the two individuals. Buber (1923/1958) described "I–Thou" encounter, which he saw as full and open intimate contact, with each recognising the humanity, uniqueness, relatedness, and separateness of the other. He said it is in such relating that we ourselves become fully human and can experience God. In comparison, "I–It" relating is our everyday relating to objects, which is at times necessary and efficient, but at worst can be distancing, exploitative, alienating, or objectifying.

Tillich

Another theologian renowned for his existential thinking was German-born Protestant, Paul Tillich (1886–1965), who left for the US in the 1930s and later became tutor to the existentialist psychologist, Rollo May (who, in turn, inspired Eric Berne). Tillich (1952) rejected the idea of a personal God but said that God was a symbol of the reality of life and was manifested in human beings. He distinguished between "neurotic anxiety" and the "existential anxiety" of our non-being, saying we needed to face and accept our non-being in order to embrace fully our being and live a full life.

Jaspers and Marcel

A welcome message of hope in relationality was brought by the German psychiatrist and philosopher, Karl Jaspers (1883–1969), and the French philosopher and playwright, Gabriel Marcel (1889–1973). Jaspers (1925/1960) emphasised the redemptive power of communication and stressed the importance of focusing on the transcendental aspects of our existence rather than our everyday preoccupations. He said our limitations remind us of our existence: death, guilt, doubt, failure, judgement, and that we need a "worldview" (our own intellectual perspective on the world and universe) to help us not fall into despair. Marcel's message was about having faith in harmony and hope in the mystery of existence, unlike other 20th-century French existentialists such as Sartre, de Beauvoir, and Camus who believed that life is ultimately meaningless. Marcel (1964) focused on the importance of openness to others, urging humans to have fidelity to ourselves, to life and to each other, whatever the future holds.

Sartre

Hope was not the message of the 20th-century French existentialists! Jean-Paul Sartre, Simone de Beauvoir, and Albert Camus were far more pessimistic about the absurdities of life, freedom, alienation, and nothingness. Jean-Paul Sartre (1905–1980), philosopher, playwright, and political activist, was inspired by the phenomenology of Husserl and Heidegger and coined the term "existentialism" when pioneering the existentialism movement. Sartre (1943/1956) said that the nothingness at the core of human existence gives us freedom to make choices and take responsibility for our life's "project". He said that humans are "condemned to be free": we are solely responsible for determining our essence and our meaning in life through the choices and actions we take, and that having such responsibility when there is no certainty of outcome in an unfair and "absurd" world creates fear and anguish. He said that people believe in determinism (that events are determined by God or previous causes) as a defence against this freedom, which causes people to live in self-deception, inauthenticity, or "bad faith".

Camus

Much of Sartre's thinking was shared by Albert Camus (1913–1960), the French novelist and political activist. He did not describe himself as a philosopher but his writing influenced the Existentialist movement. Camus (1942/1955) said that existence is meaningless and that individuals need to embrace this meaninglessness rather than trying to escape it through outside sources such as religion (entering into "bad faith"). He described the paradoxical concept of "the absurd": we accept that we cannot find meaning in existence but we always search for it. The more hopeful message was that if we can engage with the struggle and gain awareness of the absurd and our mortality we can create meaning and a greater appreciation of life.

de Beauvoir

Simone de Beauvoir (1908–1986), philosopher, existential novelist, and feminist, was Sartre's intellectual and romantic partner. De Beauvoir (1948, 1977) inspired the second, third, and fourth wave of the feminist movement and gave a feminist slant to existence preceding essence: "One is not born but becomes a woman". She distinguished between sex and gender and argued that women's gender is a social and historical construct that has been defined in relation to men. She encouraged women to assert their free will, individual choice, and authority to become what and who they are in authenticity. She emphasised the importance of collaboration (which Sartre eventually accepted as an alternative to competition).

Merleau-Ponty

Maurice Merleau-Ponty (1908–1961), the French philosopher and phenomenologist, developed Husserl's notion of intersubjectivity by emphasising the embodied nature of human existence. Merleau-Ponty (1945/1962) believed that there is no real separation between the self and other, and said that our lives will improve if we stop objectifying and separating ourselves from our experience in the world.

From existential philosophy to existential psychotherapy

The fear and anxiety created by the Second World War led to greater receptivity to existential ideas, which were spread from Europe to the USA and Israel when great thinkers such as Tillich, Arendt, Reich, and Buber fled persecution (van Deurzen, 2012). From the middle of the 20th century, this enabled the integration of existential philosophical and phenomenological ideas into psychiatric and psychotherapeutic practice. I offer you a summary of the main developments but a fuller account of the history of existentialism and existential psychotherapy can be found in Cooper (2017) and van Deurzen (2012).

Daseinsanalysis

The first systemic existential psychotherapy was developed in the early 1940s by the Swiss psychiatrists Ludwig Binswanger (1881–1966) (a colleague of Carl Jung and a friend of Freud), and Medard Boss (1903–1990) (a mentee of Martin Heidegger). Influenced by existential-phenomenological philosophers Kierkegaard, Husserl, Heidegger, and Buber, they developed Daseinsanalysis, or "existential analysis". They emphasised a holistic understanding of human existence and psychopathology, believing that the human being could only be understood in the totality of his or her existence (their "being-in-the-world"). They believed that a supportive reflective space to explore the client's experiences through description rather than interpretation could help people "open up" to others and their world and rediscover their spirit, passion and enthusiasm for life and authenticity in living.

Existential psychoanalysis and psychiatry

A philosophical understanding and critique of psychiatry was furthered by the German psychiatrist and philosopher, Karl Jaspers (1883–1969) and the libertarian and moral philosopher, Thomas Szasz (1920–2012), who moved to the US from Budapest in 1938. Szasz criticised the social control of psychiatry and psychiatric diagnosis, suggesting that it was a socio-political construct designed to mystify experience and reduce people's freedom and responsibility. Meanwhile, an existential approach to psychoanalysis was developed by the German Jewish philosopher and psychoanalyst, Erich Fromm (1900–1980), who moved to the US in 1934 and integrated social, political, spiritual, psychological, and philosophical ideas into his psychoanalytic writing and work. Fromm (1957) saw the attempts to escape our psychological and personal freedom and subsequent responsibilities as the root of all psychological conflicts. He wrote about the importance of love as interpersonal creativity, distinguishing it from notions of romantic love, which he saw as pathological. In the UK, the German–Jewish psychoanalyst, Hans Cohn (1916–2004), developed an interest in Heideggerian existentialism and became editor of *Existential Analysis*, the journal of the Society for Existential Analysis.

Meaning-centred therapies

One of the treasures that came out of the atrocities of the Second World War was the influential work of the Austrian–Jewish psychiatrist, Viktor Frankl (1905–1997). He conceived his own existential psychotherapy ("logotherapy" or "meaning therapy") whilst incarcerated at Auschwitz during the holocaust (where his family were tragically exterminated). Frankl (1946/1969) believed that finding purpose and meaning in life is the central human motivation (as opposed to Freud's "pleasure" and Adler's "power"), and that extreme psychological distress can result when people cannot find meaning in crisis. He saw that people then attempt to fill the existential vacuum of meaninglessness with self-destructive behaviours such as addictions, compulsions, and phobias. Logotherapy helps people discover renewed meaning and purpose by exploring the, often unconscious, things in their lives that feel intrinsically meaningful to them. Logotherapy was continued in Canada by the Chinese-born logotherapist, Paul Wong (1937–), who founded the Meaning-Centred Counselling Institute.

Existential-humanistic psychotherapy

In the US in the 1950s, the integration of existential and humanistic ideas led to Carl Rogers' and Abraham Maslow's humanistic psychology movement and the transition from existential psychiatry and psychoanalysis into existential-humanistic psychotherapy by Rollo May (1909–1994). Together with Ernst Angel and Henri Ellenberger, May edited the ground-breaking book, *Existence* (1958), which influenced James Bugental (1915–2008) and Irvin Yalom (1931–). Bugental (1981) focused on the nature and value of therapeutic presence as a way of helping people live more authentically and responsibly. He had a more experiential approach, focusing on bodily and affective experiences and intrapsychic dynamics, while Yalom's "existential psychodynamics" is more analytical and interpretative. Yalom used theories of resistance, transference, and unconscious processes to understand an individual's mental misery in terms of problematic interactions with others (Cooper, 2017). Drawing on Kierkegaard and Nietzsche's individualism and the aloneness of humans in facing their anxiety of existence, Yalom (1980) outlined the four givens of human existence: death, isolation, freedom/responsibility, and meaninglessness (while Bugental (1981) added a fifth: confronting embodiment). The social and spiritual arenas were included in an existential-integrative approach by the American existential-humanistic psychologist, Kirk Schneider (1956–). Using Eye movement desensitisation and reprocessing (EMDR), Acceptance and Commitment Therapy (ACT) and his "awe-based" practice, Schneider (2008) aimed for "setting people free".

Existential-phenomenological approach

The charismatic, influential and divisive Scottish psychiatrist and psychoanalyst, R.D. Laing (1927–1989), brought the existential-phenomenological approach to Europe in the 1960s and 1970s. Influenced by Sartre's socio-political thinking, he advocated using ground-breaking philosophical methods, rather than medical ones, for treating schizophrenia and "ontological insecurity" (lack of sense of self or "being"). Laing (1960) ensured the political, family, and early traumatic context was considered when trying to understand the meaning and communication of psychotic symptoms, and aimed to humanise the psychiatric system and reduce alienation of patients by breaking down the power of psychiatrists and their objectification of patients. He advocated a phenomenological approach, staying with the client's lived experience at a descriptive level rather than interpretative. Buber's work on "I–Thou" encounter, authenticity and genuineness inspired him to create a movement of therapeutic communities to offer emotionally unstable people an alternative to psychiatric care and an "awakening to love" (Gans, 2015). In a parallel with the Schiffs in TA, his radical and unconventional methods, plus sometimes questionable boundaries, led to him being ostracised by the psychiatric community. However, his influence is still felt in the contemporary existential-phenomenological psychotherapy field. He inspired the moral and ethical work of Aaron Esterson (1923–1999) (Laing & Esterson, 1964), Peter Lomas' (1924–2010) focus on the therapeutic relationship being both very special and intensely ordinary (Lomas, 1981), and the "British School of Existential Therapy" (Cohn, 1997; van Deurzen & Adams, 2016; Du Plock, 1997; Spinelli, 2015).

This is now referred to as the European Existential-phenomenological approach (van Deurzen & Adams, 2016). They emphasise Heidegger's "being-in-the-world-with-others" nature of human existence rather than the individualism of other more humanistic approaches. Cooper (2017) outlines two different strands to existential-phenomenological therapy:

Philosophical existential-phenomenological therapy, based on the work of *Emmy van Deurzen* (1951–), a Netherlands-born existential therapist, psychologist, philosopher, and writer, who founded the first existential therapy training programme in the UK at Regent's College (now University), the New School of Psychotherapy and Counselling in London, and the Society for Existential Analysis and its journal in 1988. Van Deurzen (2012) uses existential philosophical ideas to support clients to accept the limitations and paradoxes of being, while moving towards more engaged, inspired, and meaningful ways of being in the fourfold dimensions of life: physical, personal, social/cultural, and spiritual.

Relational existential-phenomenological therapy, based around the work of *Ernesto Spinelli* (1949–), an Italian-born British psychotherapist, who trained as a psychologist in Canada and the UK and collaborated with van Deurzen at Regent's College. Influenced by Carl Rogers and the US humanistic-existential tradition, Spinelli (2015) emphasises the therapeutic relationship, working descriptively, and conceptualising clients' experiences from an intersubjective standpoint rather than on the unconscious and intrapsychic dynamics of psychoanalytic thinking.

Existential perspectives in Berne's TA

Intuition and phenomenology

Eric Berne was developing his thinking around TA at the same time as the rise of existential psychotherapy, and was particularly influenced by Kierkegaard and May. He encouraged TA trainees to familiarise themselves with existential psychotherapy (Berne, 1961, pp. 84–85) and viewed TA as a "systematic phenomenology" (Berne, 1961, p. 270). The existential-phenomenological psychotherapist, Simon Du Plock, sees the significance of intuition in phenomenology, describing it as "a method of investigating the world in which all prejudice and assumptions are put aside in order to meet the world directly through intuition" (Du Plock, 1997, p. 5). Berne's (1977) early studies on intuition, and thus phenomenology, in the medical corps of the US army were instrumental in the development of TA and ego state theory (Berne, 1961).

Philosophical principles of TA

Berne's philosophical principles of TA were also "within a humanistic/existential framework of values" (Clarkson, 1992, p. 1), encompassing personal responsibility, freedom to choose, thrownness, and aloneness. Berne communicated these existential ideas through the symbolism of poker:

> Now here's what I mean by existential: Everybody's on their own. Nobody's going to feel sorry for you. You're fully responsible for everything you do. Once you put the money in the pot, you've put it in the pot. You can't blame anybody else. You have to take the consequences of that. There's no copping out.
> (Berne, 1971, p. 8)

His decisional philosophy shares a desire with existential psychotherapy to explore how we are limiting our present life by our past choices, which enables us to make new decisions to face an uncertain future with greater resilience, openness and freedom of choice and responsibility about how we want to live (van Deurzen & Adams, 2016). For Berne (1964), we could see this as movement from script into autonomy.

Life positions

Berne hinted at the existential universality of the human condition in his four life positions which he said were "universal among all mankind, because all mankind nurses at his mother's breast and gets the message there" (Berne, 1966, p. 87). He believed we start life in an authentic relational "I'm OK, You're OK" position, which values self and other in our humanity and which we could equate to Sartre's concept of pure innocence and intentionality (Nuttall, 2006).

Clarkson (1992, p. 14) suggests these life positions were about "valuing self and others in the existential knowledge of our tragic 'thrownness'" (Heidegger, 1927/1999): we are thrown together with the universal givens of existence that were present before birth and will be so after death. Existentially, all the other life positions we may visit (I'm not OK and/or You're not OK) represent ways in which we are fallen or living in "bad faith" or inauthenticity.

Four forces of human destiny

Berne's four forces of human destiny (1972/1992, cited in Nuttall, 2006) described human existence as a combination of existential givens and personal agency: the Daemon (destructive parental programming); Physis (the force of life, constructive parental programming); Fate (external forces) and Independent aspirations. Berne (1947/1968) adopted the concept of physis from Greek philosophy and from Heidegger, who referred to physis as a "power" (Heidegger, 1935/1987, p. 14) representing "Being": "Physis means the emerging and the arising, the spontaneous unfolding that lingers" (Heidegger, 1935/1987, p. 61). Berne considered it "the growth force of nature" (Berne, 1947/1969, p. 369), an existential approach which Du Plock asserted "is grounded in a view of the human being as constantly changing, flexible and always in the process of becoming" (Du Plock, 1997, p. 4). This has been illustrated by the expanding, pulsating integrating Adult (Tudor, 2003), and Tudor and Summers thus suggest that co-creative TA is "essentially a phenomenological and existential process" (Tudor & Summers, 2014, p. 64). Whilst the shared responsibility and authenticity of the two-person co-creative approach is in tune with existential psychotherapy, Tudor and Summers do not advocate the "bracketing" of the phenomenological approach, but propose full use of the therapist's self and subjectivity in present-centred relating. Whether it can be truly described as a phenomenological approach is therefore debatable.

Limits of existentialism in TA

Whilst Berne clearly was influenced by existentialism, he was also influenced by his medical and psychoanalytic background and therefore much of his thinking was at odds with the existential approach. Whilst we can link some of his theories to existential ideas (Nuttall, 2006), Berne often did not do so explicitly. More than that, his thinking around script, games, ego states and transactions, as well as his use of terms such as "diagnosis", "cure", and "treatment planning", was often pathologising and reductionist, rather than seeing individuals in terms of their whole existence. His method was interpretative, a one-person psychology (Stark, 2000), and his views on cure had a grandiosity about them that does not honour the existential approach: "There's only one paper to write which is called 'How to Cure Patients' – that's the only paper that's really worth writing if you're really going to do your job" (Berne, 1971, p. 12).

His concept of script cure is in contrast to van Deurzen-Smith's (1990, p. 161) perspective of the existential therapist who "resists the temptation to change the client". Berne (1957) mentioned the concept of "Thanatos" (the Freudian death instinct), but did not fully address the fact that death and suffering cannot be changed, only accepted and embraced. Tragically, and somewhat ironically, Berne died prematurely, death being the ultimate existential given he could not cure.

Berne's autonomy can be linked to the authenticity of the existential approach (which I address in the next chapter), but his views were contradictory and his writing on intimacy and authenticity were extremely limited. It was left to Petruska Clarkson (1995) to bring into TA the intimacy of Buber's (1923/1958) "I–Thou" relating as one of her five forms of the therapeutic relationship (the "I–You" relationship). Heiller & Sills' (2010) beautiful chapter on an existential perspective to life script showed how script can be seen as an existential striving for meaning-making, but little has been developed since then regarding an existential approach to TA. This is where this book comes in! In subsequent chapters I attempt to take TA back to its existential roots, challenge some of the inconsistencies, and develop some of Berne's existential thinking to show how we can truly integrate an existential perspective into a relational transactional analysis.

The individuality and uniqueness of existential perspectives

How each practitioner does this is dependent on their unique personal style, which brings us full circle back to our philosophical values. Van Deurzen sums up the diversity of existential psychotherapy, thought and practice in her description of it as "a philosophical therapy, which is practised in as many different ways as there are existential therapists" (Van Deurzen, 2012, p. 12). This sounds remarkably similar to the beautiful diversity of TA practitioners! Like any relational approach to psychotherapy, we can view existential therapy as an attitude or stance rather than as a separate modality, which gives us significant freedom to be creative and decide for ourselves how we want to practice from an existential perspective. This is why existentialism is such a great philosophy to integrate into TA.

There is not one objective truth, no certainty, no one right way to be a psychotherapist, consultant, supervisor, or teacher: we can listen to the diverse great minds, observe the tutors, supervisors, therapists, and writers who inspire us, think about our work through the lens of philosophies, methodologies, and theories, challenge our unthought-through assumptions, carefully consider ethical principles ... and then decide for ourselves. We should not just follow the crowd (Kierkegaard) or have a herd mentality (Nietzsche). Long gone is the idea advocated by Berne that one transactional analyst could replace another mid-therapy and the client would not notice the difference! Existential thought and wisdom enable us to find our own "truth", beliefs, values, creativity, and individuality, not someone else's. We are unique and will always bring a truly individual personal style to our therapeutic relationships that is unlike anyone else's: just like human existence itself. Is this not something to celebrate and get excited about? I think so!

Alongside this individuality, I see some themes and practices that are common to all existential practitioners:

- Being genuine, authentic and direct with our clients, rather than being a "blank screen"
- Exploring the dilemmas, difficulties, and tensions in life
- Helping our clients acknowledge, accept, and learn from guilt, anxiety, despair, and disturbance
- Grappling with the human givens of existence, encouraging our clients to acknowledge and act on their freedom and responsibility
- Talking about death and making meaning of life
- Helping people grow, develop, and flourish by becoming more authentic, and living more in accordance with their true values and beliefs
- Recognising the adult has a developmental process: "we are becoming, not ever become"
- Exploring all interconnected aspects of our clients' past, present, and future, their being (emotions, thoughts, beliefs, behaviours, physiological/embodied responses), their being-with-others (relationality), and their being-in-the-world (their holistic context, culture, spiritual life and intersectional identity in the world)

How we put this into practice is going to be different for different practitioners, with each individual client, and at different stages of our career. I offer some dilemmas of existential practice (Cooper, 2017) to give food for thought about your personal style.

- Are you more authentic and real or a blank screen?
- Are you more directive or non-directive?
- Are you more explanatory and interpretative or enquiring and descriptive?
- Are you seeking to explore pathology or rather seeking health and to de-pathologise?
- Are you more challenging or more supportive?
- Are you more technique-based or non-technique-based?
- Are you more orientated to the here-and-now (immediacy) or to events and relationships outside the therapy room?
- Are you more philosophically orientated or psychologically orientated?
- Are you more about accepting our aloneness and isolation in life or encouraging connection and relationality?
- Are you more about accepting the meaninglessness of life or about making meaning?

- Are you about bracketing your subjectivity or using it to explore the intersubjective?
- Are you wanting to seek knowledge and certainty or accept uncertainty?
- Are you more about accepting the individuality of life or the universality of life?
- Do you see therapy and consultative work as about accepting suffering and despair or about embracing hope and optimism?

As you read this book, I encourage you to reflect on how the way you work with each of these poles of existential practice is guided by your philosophical values of life. If your methodology, practice and theories are truly in line with these values and beliefs, you will be living and working with authenticity. This is the focus of the next chapter and is what I believe is critical to our work, as well as foundational to an existential approach to TA.

Chapter 2

Authenticity, alienation, and encounter

Our individual philosophical life values will guide our preferred personal style of psychotherapy, teaching and consultation. With authenticity as one of my key philosophical values, it is no wonder that I embrace the existential perspective, as a striving for authenticity is at the root of the existential approach. The word "authentic" is derived from "*authentes*" (ancient Greek for "authority; authorship"), and "*authentikos*" ("real, genuine"). Growing in authenticity is therefore twofold: it is about actively and creatively taking responsibility for becoming the author of our own lives and, in so doing, becoming increasingly real and genuine in relationship with ourselves, others, and the world. As we become increasingly real, we can claim further authorship of our lives and so our authenticity flourishes in ever-expanding spirals. In this chapter, I suggest that it is the offering of our authentic self in genuine relationship with our clients that invites them into authentic and intimate encounter. This may help to relieve alienation, aid our clients in becoming more fully themselves, and enable us to take greater responsibility for our lives, beliefs and values.

Authenticity, autonomy, and transactional analysis (TA)

Authenticity, integrity, and intimate encounter (and thus an existential perspective) are foundational to TA. As Berne said,

> Insofar as actual living in the world is concerned, transactional analysis shares with existential analysis a high esteem for and a keen interest in, the personal qualities of honesty, integrity, autonomy and authenticity, and their most poignant social manifestations in encounter and intimacy.
>
> (Berne, 1966, p. 305)

He suggested that the aim of psychotherapy was "autonomy" (Berne, 1964): increasing our existential capacity for awareness, spontaneity, and intimacy, and claiming freedom, responsibility, and power in life. "Each person designs his own life. Freedom gives him the power to carry out his own designs, and power gives him the freedom to interfere with the designs of others" (Berne,

DOI: 10.4324/9781003475217-4

1972/1992, in Nuttall, 2006, p. 220). For Berne, the negative power of others over us in early life (and reinforced by later experiences) is what creates the unhelpful and unconscious messages and beliefs of our life script, turning the "prince or princess into a frog" (Berne, 1972/1992). For Berne, this limiting script creates the story of our lives and relationships, diminishes our autonomy, and, out of awareness, leads us to discount our freedom and responsibility for our own lives. From this perspective, script effectively "militates against people's ability to take responsibility for themselves…and their own growth and well-being" (Clarkson, 1992, p. 6). From an existential stance, unconscious adaptations of script therefore mean we live inauthentically and are thus alienated from ourselves, others and the world.

Unfortunately, Berne's (1961) psychoanalytic striving for "cure" from script (turning the frog back into the prince or princess) by "diagnosing" and "treating" the client's pathology through decontamination and deconfusion work provided an ongoing tension to his fundamental existential perspective. In the later years of his life, he became increasingly pessimistic in his outlook, focusing less on the health of autonomy and more on the pathology and inauthenticity of script and games (Berne, 1964). However, he still viewed games from an existential outlook, describing them as the unconscious and unhelpful relational interactions that help people defend against their existential anxiety and a need for security and certainty. He promoted the concept of intimacy in both his theories of autonomy and as the "end goal" of time-structuring (Berne, 1964), describing it as "candid, game-free relationship, with mutual free giving and receiving and without exploitation" (Berne, 1972, p. 115), yet his medicalised approach was the antithesis to intimacy. Berne used illustrations such as straightening the "bent pennies" (Berne, 1961) and "removing the splinter" (Berne, 1971) that equated the therapist with a medical doctor, advocating for quick cure in four stages (social control, symptomatic relief, transference cure, and script cure) and even suggesting the possibility of a one-session cure. In this, he completely missed the opportunity to attend to the inevitable struggles, tensions, and suffering of life and humanity.

Some of Berne's colleagues suggested that he personally had difficulties with intimacy, and we must wonder whether his medicalised approach sadly gave him the psychological distance in relationship that he needed. Steiner – Berne's friend and colleague – suggests Berne was not receptive to caring concern: "The distance he kept from those who loved him, and whom he loved, including myself, prevented us from comforting him" (Steiner, 1974, p. 19). Karpman, another friend and colleague of Berne's, talked about intimacy as Berne's "unfinished symphony", saying he mentioned it often but offered "no plan as to how to get there" (Karpman, 2010, p. 224). We will never know whether Berne might have finished this symphony if he had not died tragically so prematurely, but in drawing on the existential approach to authenticity and encounter, I am attempting to add another movement to his powerful incomplete composition.

What is authenticity?

I think of the existential perspective to authenticity as "autonomy plus": acknowledging, in a way that is limited in the concept of autonomy, our "holistic-being-in-the-world" (Spinelli, 2005) and the "fourfold encounters of life" – physical, social/cultural, personal, and spiritual (van Deurzen & Arnold-Baker, 2018). In many ways I prefer the concept of authenticity to that of autonomy, as the 1960s Western perspective to autonomy denotes individualism and ego-centricity, alienating a large proportion of the world (much of Asia, Central and Southern America, and Africa) who prioritise family and community needs over the individual. It also does not account for connection with our bodies, the environment, the world, or the transpersonal (which I previously refer to as "our spiritual and existential search for meaning in life and our need for belonging and connection with something beyond ourselves" (Cook, 2022, p. 280)).

Some TA authors have talked about "homonomy" as an additional concept to autonomy (Massey, 2007; Tudor, 2011). This biological term was integrated into psychology by the Hungarian–American psychiatrist, Andras Angyal (1941), who described it as a focus on the dynamic and holistic entity of the person, and the interconnectedness and mutual influence of the individual, interpersonal, social, and physical environments. Whilst I appreciate the move towards a more holistic and collectivist perspective in TA, I am not a fan of the word, which cannot be found in most dictionaries! It also does not account fully for many existential givens of life. I therefore prefer to think about us aiming more simply for connection and inter-connection: with self, other, our culture, the environment, the wider world, our existence, and the transpersonal. From an existential perspective we can think about this as authenticity in a number of different contexts.

Being true to ourselves

Perhaps the most fundamental way existentialists think about authenticity is about facing the world with a sense of wonder and being true to ourselves and our beliefs, values and ideals: an "openness to Being" (Heidegger, 1927/2010). To be authentic is to be able to question and dialogue with others in order that we can gain our own understanding of life and ourselves, rather than following the crowd (Kierkegaard, 1844/1980) or herd (Nietzsche, 1886/1989). When we are truly authentic, we can think and behave for ourselves in the moment, despite uncertainty over the outcome or fears about whether we will get it "right" or whether others will agree with us. We will have more freedom from the internalised, often unconscious demands of script. Kierkegaard (1844/1980) went further, advocating for us to find a love and truth in aloneness. I see this aspect of authenticity as having similarities with Berne's "awareness": having full connection with ourselves and the wider world in the here-and-now, being free from the prejudices, biases, and contaminations of the Parent ego state and the archaic Child confusions. When one of my newly single clients was psychologically paralysed through fear of doing things on her own because of what others would think of her, she said it was not necessarily the explorations into her Parent and Child ego states that eventually made the difference, but inquiries and confrontations about how *she* wanted to live her life. Yes, others might judge her but did she want to be bound by that? Did she want to abdicate that power over her own life? How uplifting it was when she sent me a postcard from a London gallery, celebrating her newfound independence and creativity!

Being spontaneous and creative

Greater awareness releases our natural life force or "physis" (Berne, 1968) and a greater potential for more spontaneous, curious, intuitive, playful, and creative living, as well as for facing the inevitable disappointments, tensions, or tragedies of life. We have freedom to have adventures, experiment with new experiences and tolerate the anxiety of disturbance and uncertainty when making changes in our lives, trying something new, or becoming increasingly intimate in relationship. Laing saw this spontaneity as an "awakening to love" (Gans, 2015). It is when I am living authentically that I often find myself thinking and saying, "I feel really alive". I think of the aliveness I feel when facilitating tutor groups through their psychotherapy training. At some point in the year, I always ask myself why I do this job: it is disturbing, distressing, pushes me to my limits, stirs my deepest insecurities and frailties. I, along with my students, inevitably encounter the most unbearable aspects of humanity: grief, terror, cruelty, oppression, contempt, hate, envy, shame, embarrassment, and destruction. There is often grief and anger when someone does not reciprocate, wounds us when we have been vulnerable, or leaves prematurely and unexpectedly. And yet throughout the year, we also expand our capacity for intimacy, sharing our vulnerabilities, being accepted for our fallible humanity, laughing and crying together, learning from each other, joyfully celebrating each other's achievements, grieving the final goodbye. Those of us who have been courageous in our vulnerability – myself included – have had the opportunity to creatively experience group and others' presence in a way that enables greater honesty, disturbance, spontaneity, playfulness, maturity in love, and authenticity. We have become more enlivened; we feel more truly and creatively alive.

Being connected with others

Such intimacy or "presence" is how many existentialists describe authenticity: the capacity for fidelity, availability and receptivity to the Other (Marcel, 1964), or an openness to acceptance or forgiveness (Tillich, 1952). Buber counteracts the individualism of philosophers such as Kierkegaard by urging us to find authenticity in reciprocal relationship: "the inmost growth of the self is not accomplished, as people like to suppose today, in man's relation to himself, but in the relation between one and the other" (Buber, 1923/1958, p. 61). He saw the connection with God (the "eternal Thou" or "Centre") emerging through authenticity in intimate "I–Thou" relating, which I expand on later.

Facing existential anxiety

Authenticity can also be about facing existential anxiety, our "Being-towards-death" (Heidegger, 1927/2010), and thus taking greater responsibility for making choices that enable a more vibrant, vital and meaningful existence. In TA, anxiety has often been seen as pathologically script-based: a "racket" or substitute feeling (English, 1971) covering split-off anger, sadness or fear, or signalling introjected Parent/Child relational units (Little, 2006) that represent longings for and fears of intimacy because of an unsupported traumatic history or an anxious care-giver. Whilst of course we need to help our clients with symptomatic relief from unmanageable anxiety and to explore unconscious processes surrounding the anxiety, some anxiety is a normal and healthy part of authentic human existence. Anxiety about our mortality is inevitable and we need to help our clients tolerate and act upon it rather than too quickly seeking to soothe – perhaps in an attempt to soothe ourselves. Too often we attempt to drown out our death anxiety with the "noise and confusion" (Kierkegaard, 1844/1980) of overwork, addictions, phobias, obsessions, and the like, rather than facing with courage the anxiety of our nonbeing and thus gaining a sense of autonomy, self-actualisation, and authenticity (Tillich, 1952). As Kierkegaard (1844/1980, p. 155) said: "Whoever has learned to be anxious in the right way has learned the ultimate". I focus on this in later chapters.

Facing existential guilt

Failing to taking responsibility for choosing the direction of our lives and not fulfilling our potential can mean we experience existential guilt. TA practitioners often too quickly attempt to alleviate a client's guilt, seeing it simply as an unhealthy "I'm not OK, you're OK" life position (Berne, 1962/1976), or a "racket" feeling covering authentic anger, blame, loss, fear, or sadness. It may be, but it may also be an important sign to us that we are not living authentically. Kierkegaard suggested that "the more profoundly guilt is discovered, the greater the genius" (Kierkegaard, 1844/1980, p. 109). Existential guilt is often revealed to us through our conscience and dreams (Heidegger, 1927/2010). When I was contemplating whether I could make the time to write this book, I dreamt about a much-loved client who was a very competent psychotherapy trainee struggling psychologically with the concept of starting work in private practice. In my dream I stopped at a service station mid-journey, to be met by my client serving fried chicken and fries, resplendent in slightly incongruent (for the eatery) chef whites! In my dream, I was disappointed that they were wasting their significant therapeutic capabilities and challenged them, before leaving with renewed determined to write my book. Discussing the dream with my client led to fruitful conversations about previously unformulated fears and regrets, the decisions they were making, what was stopping them fulfilling their potential, the incongruence they felt, and their responsibilities for their life. I also saw it as a strong communication to myself to make the time to write this book, for which I am clearly now taking responsibility!

Finding meaning in absurdity

In order to accomplish our "projects", we need to make "a decisive dedication to what we want to accomplish for our lives" (Hoffman, 1993, p. 229). Making meaning out of our life in order to live authentically takes commitment, drive, ambition, perseverance, and a sense of humour at the "absurdity" or apparent meaninglessness of life. Sartre (1943/1956) described it as the authenticity of commitment to one's own projects in the face of this meaninglessness. In the absurdity of life, we are like the mythological Sisyphus who was condemned by the Greek gods to roll a rock to the top of a mountain, which repeatedly rolls back down (Camus, 1942/1955). Despite this absurdity, Sisyphus did not give up and gained the strength and dignity to ascend and descend the mountain with joy as well as sorrow. Helping people integrate both the joy and sorrow of an authentic life, and finding their life's meaning, is the "life project" of psychotherapy. This, for me, helps me live more authentically as it gives my life meaning. As Frankl says: "the meaning of life is to help others find the meaning of theirs" (Frankl, 1946/1969, p. 165).

Inauthenticity and alienation

We cannot help people live more authentically without considering the factors that lead to inauthenticity or "bad faith" (Sartre, 1943/1956). For Berne, this was the impact of an individual's life script; for the radical psychiatry movement (Steiner et al., 1975), it was the alienation caused by social, cultural, and political oppression. Steiner described alienation as "a condition in which people are estranged from their powers" (Steiner, 1979, p. 95), and "a feeling within a person that he is not part of the human species, that she is dead or that everyone is dead, that he does not deserve to live, or that someone wishes her to die" (Steiner, 1979, p. 11). Alienation is a foundational concept for existential philosophy and psychotherapy and is considered the root cause of inauthentic living (van Deurzen & Kenward, 2005). It goes further than radical psychiatry in that it considers alienation in any aspect of existence: not just the social, political, economic, and cultural but also the psychological, philosophical, spiritual, and relational. Such alienation is described by the American philosopher, Allen Wood, as "a psychological or social evil, characterised by one or another type of harmful separation, disruption or fragmentation which sunders things that belong together" (Wood, 2005, p. 21). We can therefore think of it as any harmful disconnection from self, other, culture, environment, world, existence, or the transpersonal.

Alienation from self and other

Alienation from aspects of self or other can be caused, in childhood or adult life, by experiences of unsupported trauma, abuse, oppression, neglect, bullying, humiliation, abandonment, spiritual abuse, betrayal, parental alienation, chronic illness, disability, neurodivergence, and the like. We sadly see such alienation every day in our consulting rooms and in the wider world, manifested in war, relational breakdown, oppression, prejudice, depression, anxiety, lack of sense of self, narcissism, loneliness, isolation, and a sense of meaninglessness. TA offers a theoretical understanding of this alienation through such intrapsychic and interpersonal theories as ego states, script, games, transactions, and impasse theory (Goulding & Goulding, 1978; Mellor, 1980). It also provides methodologies and methods for working with alienation through therapeutic operations, decontamination, and deconfusion (Berne, 1961), and empathic transactions, the developmental model of self, and transferential dynamics (Hargaden & Sills, 2002). Plato (in Stace, 1920) considered such lack of integration or fragmentation of the self as a form of *philosophical alienation* occurring as an imbalance in harmony between reason, emotion, and the senses in the psyche of the human soul (which sounds remarkably similar to the thinking, feeling, and behaviour of ego states or Erskine and Zalcman's (1979) script system).

We can also be alienated from our self through conforming to social demands – which Kierkegaard (1844/1980) described as *existential alienation* of self – or by not accepting responsibility for our freedom or true values and beliefs, as in Sartre's (1943/1956) *ethical alienation* of self. For Kierkegaard, overcoming existential alienation was through "self-becoming" and accounting for each individual's uniqueness through relation with the "Absolute" (God), whilst for Sartre it was by facing our existential anxiety, taking responsibility for our life choices, and living authentically according to our true values and beliefs.

This may sound relatively easy, but challenging long-held inauthentic beliefs and value systems can be deeply distressing. Change creates disruption, uncertainty, and anxiety (particularly when it hinges on our foundational belief system), because with every change we experience a "movement-towards-death" (Heidegger, 1927/2010). We need to let go of our old self and are uncertain about who the new self will be and how we will be impacted. This connects us to death anxiety (Spinelli, 2015). Wood (2005) suggests that, paradoxically, we can even feel a greater sense of alienation when we start to question our core beliefs:

> Reflection on your beliefs, values, or social order can also alienate you from them. It can undermine your attachment to them, cause you to feel separated from them, no longer identified with them... they are yours, but you are alienated from them.
>
> (Wood, 2005, p. 21)

We therefore need to be careful that we do not impose our agenda or beliefs and values on to our clients, risking further alienation. When I started questioning my lifelong faith, I was gripped with terror of my non-being and a sense of existential aloneness and alienation from self and God. Who was I without the same faith that had upheld me and given my life meaning? It was the relational connection with a spiritual accompanier (a "soul friend" who accompanies you on your spiritual journey) that counteracted my sense of alienation and helped me face with courage my old beliefs, questions and doubts, and think through for myself what I wanted my new beliefs and values to be.

Alienation from existence

Making choices to change such beliefs can be immeasurably difficult because of an "ontological insecurity" (Laing, 1960) or "ontological alienation" (Heidegger, 1927/2010). This ontological insecurity is the alienation from self and other emanating from a disconnection from one's being or existence, experienced as immense anxiety and a reduced capacity for personal authority, openness, discovery, and curious discourse. Laing suggests that such ontological insecurity creates an internal schizoid split between accepted and "not me" parts, and a distancing from a world that is considered dangerous and threatening to self-autonomy. Mental disturbance (such as psychosis, schizophrenia, or multiple personalities) can be a means of survival and communication of a person's fragile existential condition, but can lead to further alienation from aspects of one's self or the world. For Laing, the antidote to ontological alienation is humanisation through presence and intensity of therapeutic engagement, leading to greater spontaneity and an awakening to love.

Van Deurzen believes that "the ontological insecurity at the core of schizophrenia is essentially there in all of us" (Van Deurzen, 1998, p. 10), explaining it as "pure existential anxiety" or homesickness: the dread of nothingness and a sense of not-at-homeness at the heart of the human condition. Fromm (1955) agrees, saying that, because of the insecure and uncertain nature of existence, a sensitive, thinking and alive person cannot feel secure or certain about anything. Both agree that the antidote to alienation is therefore to find ways of courageously and constructively coming to terms with this given of existence: "The psychic task which a person can and must set for himself, *is not to feel secure, but to be able to tolerate insecurity, without panic and undue fear ...*" (Fromm, 1955, p. 196, original emphasis).

Flo

Because of significant childhood trauma and diagnosed ADHD, Flo came to therapy with a sense of "nowhereness". I got the sense of a deeply alienated soul who found it hard both to connect intimately and to differentiate between self and other. Once Flo felt trusting enough to remove the mask a little and reveal more of her core self, the disturbance of her existential insecurity started to emerge. For Flo, I was alternately the withholding, loved, fearful or envied other. With anger and deep grief, she would tell me that I was not available enough outside our twice-weekly sessions, I didn't love her enough because she would never be part of my family, I would abandon her and not think twice about her when I went on holiday. She described her fear of my eyes, often turning away from me or sitting behind a chair, and spoke of an anxiety that my attention would shatter her into millions of jagged pieces. She sometimes became hostile with envy about how she perceived my internal security, intelligence, wisdom, humour, as well as my house, family, and work. I did not attempt to alleviate these feelings, but provided the holding, support, and challenge of my engaged and containing presence that enabled her to feel safe enough to slowly communicate the indescribable grief of her soul. I was not trying to provide a new "secure base" of infancy, or protection from her anxiety, but to help her gradually tolerate the indescribable internal devastation; to embrace connection at the same time as separation; and to help Flo create her own "internal home" by enlarging her capacity for grief, mourning, and differentiation. Her newly expanded internal home was evident when she returned after a two-week break. When once my holidays felt unsurvivable for her, this time she told me about her dream that she had arrived for a therapy session, only to find me asleep in my chair. She quietly shut the door and left, happy that I was relaxing and realising that she should not intrude until it was time for me to wake up. Flo was telling me that she was better tolerating insecurity, and – even if unwanted – accepting our separation and differentiation.

Social, political, and economic alienation

Frantz Fanon, the Afro-Caribbean psychiatrist, political philosopher, and critical theorist, suggested that the Western frame of reference focuses too much on individual pathology and self-alienation, risking not accounting for cultural, social, and political context: "A normal black child, having grown up with a normal family, will become abnormal at the slightest contact with the white world" (Fanon, 1952/2008, p. 122). Fanon differentiates between different forms of alienation – from self, the significant other, the general other, one's culture, and from creative social praxis. He suggests that, whilst we are all human and have fundamentally similar human experiences, the history of alienation through colonisation, racism, and intergenerational trauma means we have very different experiences of the world in that human body. He argues that past social structures alienated both Black and White people, the privileged and the marginalised, because *both* are objectified in the process and locked in the separation of blackness or whiteness.

Of course, privilege makes objectification more bearable and provides greater possibility to move from alienation to connection. Still today, it is predominantly privileged Whites, for example, that can benefit from psychotherapy and psychoanalysis. Influenced by philosophers such as Fanon, Hegel, and Marx – who argued that capitalism alienated workers and reduced human beings to assets, liabilities, profits, and losses – the radical psychiatry movement (Steiner & Wyckoff, 1975) introduced into TA the concept of social, political, and economic alienation. They proposed that "people's troubles have their source not within them but in their alienated relationships, in their exploitation, in polluted environments, in war, and in the profit motive" (Steiner & Wyckoff, 1975, pp. 3–4) and that "all alienation is the result of oppression about which the oppressed has been mystified or deceived" (Steiner & Wyckoff, 1975, p. 11). They argued that our role as practitioners is to help bring the mystification into awareness, enable them to feel and express the anger about the oppression and deception, and find liberation and authenticity through relational contact and social and political action.

Cornell (2020) critiques Steiner's position as being too focused on the external forces of oppression and ignoring the forces of one's own unconscious: our own distorted thinking, projections, and personal vulnerabilities that may also foster malaise and alienation. Without acknowledging and exploring our unconscious processes, we risk unwittingly further oppressing and alienating our clients. This has been addressed in TA by a more relational approach to radical psychiatry and intersectionality (Baskerville, 2022; Minikin, 2018, 2023). Minikin suggests that it is the examination of co-created transferential processes and mutuality of contact in the therapeutic relationship that brings awareness to the psychic and cultural death experienced through alienation. With this awareness comes a necessary disturbance, and we need to help our clients come back to life by "[finding] the warrior, the fighter within to rouse us into a positive state of aggression and engagement with life outside and inside…socially and psychically" (Minikin, 2018, p. 122). This new connection or "awakening" to self, plus relational encounters with others, enables a capacity to tolerate and engage with difference ("plurality") and thus, I believe, greater authenticity.

Simon

When facilitating a new group's training course with experienced practitioners, the first check-in was surprisingly intimate and touching. I was fully immersed in the connection with each individual, when the group's intimacy was cut through, quite brutally, by Simon, the last man to check in. He said he had had enough of me talking and did not want to hear from me when he spoke. I felt like I had been hit violently, his words cutting through the connection and shattering the intimate atmosphere into a thousand fragmented pieces of alienation. The group froze and, as he checked in, I frantically tried to work out what had happened and how to respond. Yet I was in a double-bind: if I responded I was not respecting his request for me to be silent, which could be oppressive. If I did not respond I was left silenced, which definitely felt oppressive. I decided to share my dilemma with him, explaining calmly that I did not want to override his request, but that I felt silenced and did not want to be (and could not be as everyone there was paying me to teach them!).

The spontaneous reaction from the group still brings tears to my eyes. They collectively supported and empathised with me, whilst challenging their colleague and the gendered oppression they had witnessed. They spoke authentically of their distress at the intimacy being fractured and their subsequent wariness of him, and acknowledged the challenge for themselves of being so intimate in a new group of strangers. They finally, and movingly, returned to empathise with and support Simon so that he did not also feel alienated from the group. The mutuality of contact and conflict helped to bring alienation into awareness which enabled our engagement with the emerging disturbance. Simon and I talked about the impact on each other: my feeling of alienation as a woman being silenced by a man (which was not unfamiliar to me), and his schizoid fears of the intimacy taking him by surprise, as well as my authenticity and power being too much for him. He realised he defensively maintained distance and control by attacking the person in power, but ultimately resulting in further alienation of self and other, which was not what he really desired.

Shortly after I wrote this section, I read this extract from Laing's *The Divided Self*, which made me think of this encounter with Simon:

> the person whom we call "schizoid" feels both more exposed, more vulnerable to others than we do, and more isolated. Thus, a schizophrenic may say that he is made of glass, of such transparency and fragility that a look directed at him splinters him to bits and penetrates straight through him. We may suppose that precisely as such he experiences himself.
>
> (Laing, 1960, p. 38)

How apt that I described above that I had experienced Simon's schizoid process as "shattering the intimacy into a thousand fragmented pieces of alienation". Through our encounter I think we both discovered a better understanding of our unconscious processes, a greater toleration of difference, and gained increased authenticity by piecing together some of the fragments of connection caused by alienation.

Alienation from the world, the environment, and the transpersonal

When the world is experienced as dangerous or threatening, as it was for Simon, alienating ourselves from it is a desperate attempt to keep ourselves safe. In *Contextual Transactional Analysis*, James Sedgwick (2021) argues that "self-and-world" are inseparable. The individual is always shaped by their society's gaps and deficiencies and a relational psychotherapy must therefore consider the context of the client's "self-and-world" as well as the therapist's "self-and-world". Philosophically, we can think of ourselves as one fractal of a dynamic world and need connection with the world to have full consciousness (or autonomy or authenticity). This was described by the German philosopher, neuroscientist and psychiatrist, Georg Northoff (2018), as a "world-brain" connection rather than simply "mind-body". The separation of our consciousness from the world and from Universal consciousness is described by Hegel (1807/2016) as *dialectical alienation*. This can be seen in alienation from world events and relationships; from the spiritual, transcendent, or transpersonal connections of life; or from the natural world and environment (described by the American environmental and ecological philosopher, David Abram (1997), as the "more-than-human world").

The "more-than-human-world" gives me great existential comfort and spiritual connection through the natural world, music, and the arts. I once went alone to a moving and uplifting classical concert in a medieval cathedral, becoming wonderfully immersed in the spiritual connection I felt with the musicians, the instruments, the composer, the centuries of worshippers that had been there before and that were to come, as well as the thousands of workers who had built this magnificent building over hundreds of years, most of whom had died before they could see the fruition of their work. In the interval, I came back into my human world and checked my phone for messages. The woman next to me leant over and said: "isn't it a shame that so many people get their phones out rather than allowing themselves to stay immersed in the memory of the music?". It was a little shaming, but I was ultimately grateful for a very effective confrontation! I now make a conscious effort to stay connected and less alienated from my "more-than-human world".

Whilst I have adapted this phrase to account for the transpersonal, Abram's "more-than-human-world" focuses on the alienation that occurs when we fail to recognise and acknowledge how entwined we are with other animals, plants, ecosystems, and "earthly nature" that sustain us. The development of eco-TA (Barrow & Marshall, 2020, 2023) has given TA a welcome focus on this interconnection with the natural environment. Barrow and Marshall describe this as "an approach for understanding the human and the more-than-human experience that is forged in connection with the ecological context in which it occurs..." and talk about "...the agency of both human and the more-than-human partners in the encounter" (Barrow & Marshall, 2023, p. 6). Whilst eco-TA does not consider explicitly the transpersonal, I think the ecological and the spiritual are inextricably linked. In my experience, many people experience through nature a deep spiritual connection with the universe, a higher power or their God, to something greater than "I". This can help them feel part of something beyond themselves and find meaning in life and death. I am drawn to Tudor's integration into TA of the spiritual and environmental in a two-person-plus psychology, where he suggests we "pay attention to the client's sense of connection with and/or disconnection from her or his world … including relationships with her or his faith, ancestors, and natural environment (e.g., land, river, and mountains)" (Tudor, 2011, p. 53).

One of my clients found great spiritual solace when her husband was dying from cancer by walking every day in our nearby forest. She said that the trees gave her comfort, knowing that she had walked with them many times with her beloved husband, and that they would still be there once he had died, thus somehow still connecting her with him. It reminded me of Berne talking about here-and-now existential awareness being about "knowing that the trees will still be there after he dies, so [wanting] to experience them now with as much poignancy as possible" (Berne, 1964, pp. 159–160). Spirituality is one of the tenets of our human existence (van Deurzen & Arnold-Baker, 2018) and if we do not attend to the spiritual with our clients – helping them discover their own deeper meaning to their existence – we risk further alienating them. We are socially and spiritually constructed beings, and connection with others, the world, the environment, and the transpersonal is what gives us a coherent sense of self and helps us live authentically and make meaning of the past, present and future against a backdrop of eternity (van Deurzen, 2012).

Encounter: the antidote to alienation

Coming up against each other

An essential antidote to alienation is human-to-human connection. Buber (1923/1959) describes this as "I-Thou" relating, when we can experience the transpersonal though authentic human "encounter": "When we encounter another individual truly as a person, not as an object for use, we become fully human". This is in contrast to Buber's "I-It" relating which, at best can be functional or transactional, and at worst can be depersonalising, objectifying, and alienating. Encounter is not always easy or pleasant. It involves conflict, the confrontation of each other's presence, a "summoning up" (Barrow, 2020) of the other into a new relational experience or novel perspective of their existence. And we will experience the gamut of human emotion and experience: rage, aggression, love, hate, peace, envy, fear, beauty, indifference.

Cornell (2011, citing Winnicott, 1971) suggests that some "I-It" relating is necessary through exploratory play, which he suggests is "not necessarily pleasant but represents the freedom and capacity for one to come *up against* other people and the external world in its various manifestations" (Cornell, 2011, p. 341). It is creative play with our clients that can help us find the person behind the masks. We bracket our own assumptions and preconceptions, offer an openness of being, and immerse ourselves (without pathologising) in the often deeply distressing, painful, and disturbing world of another. Such play is inclusive and integrating: "…in play an object can be destroyed and restored, hurt and mended, dirtied and cleaned, killed and brought to life, with the added achievement of ambivalence in place of splitting the object (and self) into good and bad" (Winnicott, 1989, pp. 60–61). Through coming up against each other and encountering in a different playful way our clients' physical, personal, impersonal, relational and spiritual world, we can help them feel more real and find creative growth through greater individuation, integration, and relational connection.

Matt

Matt confronted me with his rage in the first five minutes of our ther-apy. He aggressively interrupted my introductory spiel, saying "I don't care what your fucking qualifications are, I'm only here because my wife told me I had to come, and I won't be staying". I was taken aback and somewhat intimidated, a little fearful for my safety. I wondered whether my "I-It" contracting was avoiding the encounter he immediately desired, so with trepidation and potency, I ditched the spiel and met him face-to-face to "summon him up" into a new relational experience. "You don't even know me, and yet you're interrupting me and being aggressive with me. Is this your usual way of relating?" I was literally on the edge of my seat, as was Matt. He came back at me forcefully, and after some time jousting back and forth, I commented on our process, asking him what it was like for him that we were engaging in this way. He paused, sat back in his seat and said in a quieter, softer tone, "I feel safe that you're standing up to me". I saw the vulnerability underneath the façade, and softened. "It sounds like underneath the anger you're actually quite scared", I offered, to which Matt broke down in tears.

My confrontation enabled his historical and present experiences of alienation from self, other, and existence to be talked about. We inves-tigated his destructiveness, passivity, avoidance, and shame, and his rage at women that ravaged his relationships. As he felt the profound grief and fear of abandonment emanating from his mother leaving him at a young age, he realised his aggressiveness had protected him from his unmanageable ontological insecurity. He was shocked and upset when I later disclosed my initial feelings of intimidation and threat, say-ing apologetically, "I don't want to be intimidating, I don't want to be that kind of man". We talked about the kind of man that he wanted to be, and, in an attempt to highlight my own imperfect humanity and minimise his sense of shame, I disclosed my own struggles with intimi-dation that sometimes emerged when I felt particularly vulnerable. "We all have the capacity for both intimidation and love", I offered. Matt later explained that my honest confrontation of his intimidation, as well as the shared humanity of my self-disclosure, were the most significant and life-changing interactions of his therapy.

Courage and risk

Our disturbance, and gradually talking through our mutual respect, trust, acceptance, and love for each other, helped both Matt and I tolerate greater levels of intimacy. But such encounter is risky and uncertain and often means sticking our neck out and leaning into "edge moments" (Leigh, 2011). We need the courage to be vulnerable, to be prepared to re-examine our beliefs and values, and to accept our own imperfections, wounds, and the less palatable "shadow" parts of ourselves. Through the courageous risk of considered self-disclosure, present-centred relating, mutuality, honesty, directness, and openness, we offer the other a sense of reciprocity, trustworthiness, warmth, playfulness, and humour. In essence, encounter is having the courage for a deep sense of personal investment. I often recognise a moment of encounter when I am physically or psychologically "on the edge of my seat", meeting each other face-to-face in spirit as well as mind and body. It is an intensity of therapeutic engagement that awakens in both of us polarities of terror and calm, love and hate, power and powerlessness, impenetrability and vulnerability. We both risk being hurt, but the potential benefits are greater mutuality, humanisation, freedom, emancipation, responsibility, spontaneity, authenticity, and maturity of love (Biesta, 2014; Laing, 1960).

Over the last few years, I have met with around 12 of my supervisees for days of group supervision. The initial motivation was to make it worthwhile for them to travel some distance to get in-person supervision. But, having already formed a trusting relationship with each of them individually, I made a conscious decision to invite them into my home (rather than a hired space) in an attempt to increase the mutuality between us and to integrate different parts of my life and humanity. This was an act of courage: I was both more relaxed in my secure environment, yet more insecure at disclosing more of myself than usual. My hope was that the sense of "home" and the offering of my humanity and vulnerability would enable honest and authentic encounters. I have not been disappointed. The days have been beautifully vulnerable, intimate, and powerfully yet manageably disturbing. Through mutual courageous risk, we have engaged in a different way with disturbance around race, gender, sexuality, neurodivergence, intrusion, educational trauma, competition, inadequacy, and shame. "Home" provided both security and threat, evoking comfort, longings, envy, and a stark reminder of our difference. But our mutuality in vulnerability provided enough security for our inevitable ontological insecurities and projections to be brought into awareness, talked about, and accepted as part of human existence without a sense of terror or panic. As a consequence, many were able to see our own and each other's humanity in more vivid colour, and experience a stronger internal psychological sense of home because of the quality of our relating. None of this would be possible without the offering of our presence and real personhood, and it is this which is the focus of the next chapter.

Chapter 3

The quality of relating

An existential approach to TA theory, methods, and methodology

The methods and methodologies of TA

Therapeutic operations

Berne was adamant that psychotherapy was about change, a cure from pathology: "the ultimate aim of transactional analysis is structural readjustment and reintegration" (Berne, 1961, p. 246). He said this could happen through restructuring and reorganising the pathology in the client's ego states: "decontamination" of the introjected Parent ego states and contaminated Child beliefs, and "deconfusion" of the archaic, traumatically fixated Child ego states. He provided "techniques" or interventions for effecting psychotherapeutic change in the form of the somewhat medically sounding eight "therapeutic operations" (Berne, 1966), almost a surgeon's handbook of how to remove the splinter. Berne said that the first six (interrogation, specification, confrontation, explanation, illustration, and confirmation) were to be used for analysis of ego states, transactions, games, and script in the decontamination phase of therapy, whilst the last two (interpretation and crystallisation) were to be used specifically for deconfusion. For Berne (1961), these therapeutic operations would move the therapy through decontamination and deconfusion via four stages of cure: social control; symptomatic relief; transference cure; and the ultimate goal of script cure.

Empathic transactions

Therapeutic operations were updated by Barbara Clark (1991) to introduce the concept of empathy, a notion noticeably absent from Berne's writing. This was further developed by Richard Erskine, Janet Moursund, and Rebecca Trautmann (1999) in their emphasis on Integrative TA and "contact-in-relationship" through empathy, attunement, and involvement. Clark renamed the therapeutic operations "empathic transactions", a transaction in TA being a verbal or non-verbal unit of social communication consisting of both a stimulus and a response (Berne, 1972). Clark proposed that empathy should be

DOI: 10.4324/9781003475217-5

communicated in such a way that the patient's experiences are understood at a profound level. This enables an empathic bond to be established between patient and therapist, thus helping the therapist meet the patient's unmet needs and enabling deconfusion of early Child ego states. Hargaden & Sills (2001, 2002) developed Clark's thinking further, giving a relational slant to each of the eight empathic transactions. They renamed "interrogation" as the less intrusive "empathic enquiry", added "holding" as a ninth intervention (similar to Bion's (1962) "containment" or Winnicott's (1960) "holding"), and suggested that all nine could be used for both decontamination and deconfusion work; deconfusion was not a separate phase but occurred implicitly from the first moment of meeting. Hargaden and Sills described empathic transactions as "A series of complementary transactions between the Adult of the client and the therapist and complementary ulterior transactions between the client's Child and the therapist's Adult" (Hargaden & Sills, 2001, p. 33), and like Clark, believed that the consistent communication of empathy and respect eventually "makes it possible for the client to feel secure enough at an "unthought" level to revive unmet needs and suppressed developmental needs" (Hargaden & Sills, 2001, p. 33).

Co-creative empathic transactional relating

Tudor (2011) and Tudor and Summers (2014) critique empathic transactions, warning of the danger of inviting idealisation for narcissistic gain in sending ulterior messages to a client's Child ego states. Instead, they advocate "co-created empathic transactional relating" (Summers & Tudor, 2000, p. 36): present-centred, Adult-to-Adult interactions through dialogue. They argue that moving from co-transferential relating (Past I–Past You) into the mutuality of present-centred relating (Present I–Present You), expands the integrating Adult of both client and therapist and results in automatic decontamination and deconfusion of the archaic Child and introjected Parent. "This perspective shifts the therapeutic emphasis away from the treatment of ego state structures and toward an exploration of how relational possibilities are co-created on a moment-to-moment basis" (Summers & Tudor, 2000, p. 36). Whilst integrative TA focuses on the quality of empathy, attunement, and involvement of the *therapist*, co-creative TA prioritises the quality of *relationship* co-created by therapist and client.

Existential transactions: the quality of relating

In this way, co-creative TA has some similarities with the existential approach which aims to move away from technique, instead preferencing exploration, awareness, and acceptance of the unresolvable over a striving for change, cure, or autonomy. It also importantly values the *qualities* of the practitioner and the *quality* of the therapeutic or consultative relationship over any theory or method. The priority is "being with" the other in dialogue and relatedness. I was once told by students in a new tutor group that they were both pleased and apprehensive to have me as their tutor because they had heard that I was "great at theory", and this was intimidating. Bristling slightly at the slight objectification of me as a theoretician rather than as a human being, I responded with a semi-playful confrontation: "I may or may not be shit-hot at theory, but I would rather you were pleased and apprehensive because I bring my presence; that's the best thing I can offer you". We then had a useful mutual exploration of what was happening between us in the immediacy of our relating and how this helped them understand themselves better, and, to quote one of the students, "Now we were off!"

I do not want to discount TA's theories and methods as they have inspired invaluable awareness and impactful change to my ways of being and relating. It was the significant impact of TA theories on my understanding of myself and my relationships that inspired me to become a therapist. I still use it every day in my therapeutic, supervisory, and educational work and it has had an immeasurable impact on a great number of people, which then has a knock-on effect on many others. Therapeutic operations and empathic transactions can give helpful structure to reflect on our therapeutic or consultative intention: to be cognisant of why we are doing what we are doing, and to provide some ideas of how to do it. What I want to do here is offer an alternative existential perspective to therapeutic relating that can be integrated with TA's methods and methodology. I describe five essential qualities, attitudes, and transactions that enable a practitioner to focus on exploration, understanding and "being with" rather than seeking change or cure. I call these *"existential transactions"*:

1 A dialogic attitude
2 Descriptive investigation
3 Acceptance
4 Presence
5 Self-disclosure

In describing these attitudes and transactions, I will show that many of the empathic transactions are useful when relating in this way. The existential-phenomenological approach, however, has more of a focus on empathic enquiry, specification, confrontation, confirmation, illustration, and holding rather than explanation and interpretation (which can increase the power differential and elevate the practitioner into the "expert" position). Interpretation and crystallisation are something that the client does for themselves, not that the practitioner imparts on them. I also see self-disclosure as an empathic transaction in its own right, and is such an important and controversial aspect of a relational existential psychotherapy that I devote the next chapter to its exploration. My use of the word "transaction" for these qualities and attitudes was deliberated carefully, as the existential approach generally eschews methods and techniques. However, I see transactions as being inherently mutual: in TA terms, a transaction is only complete if there is a response as well as a stimulus (verbal or non-verbal, conscious, or non-conscious). In existential terms, we might think of these transactions as dialogue in the immediacy of the human encounter.

A dialogic attitude

Immediacy

Immediacy is part of a dialogic attitude and is about being able to explore together in the present moment what is happening between us and how we are relating, in order that the client can get to know and understand themselves better. It is about spontaneity, naturalness, and uniqueness in an immediate and direct human encounter (Mearns & Cooper, 2005). I find it helpful to explain at the beginning of therapy that, if they are willing, we can work with the immediacy of our relating in the present moment, offering them the possibility of an "*encounter contract*" (Cook, 2023) that "[invites] clients into present-centred relating in order that we can explore together what happens between us, share responsibility, and encourage mutuality" (Cook, 2023, p. 251). Widdowson (2008) also advocates the use of "metacommunicative transactions" for immediacy in relating: interventions that explore the here-and-now process between therapist and client. For example, "I'm feeling a little distant from you right now, is it the same for you?". Daniel Stern (2004a) argues that therapist responses that offer immediacy in the present moment are far more valuable than the theory-laden interpretations with which therapists might feel more at ease. This way of being is lost if we become directive, directional or interpretative, seek particular responses or outcomes from our clients, or focus too intently on our interventions and what we are *doing* to the other. Instead, a dialogic attitude focuses on *being with* the other in a spontaneous immediate dialogue, being truthful with ourselves and our clients, and with neither person pre-determining the focus, direction, or intention of the dialogue.

A supervisee of Indian heritage told me a lovely story about taking a taxi ride in Mumbai. She and her partner were newly in love and so immersed in each other that they had been driving for some time before they realised that neither of them had told the driver where they wanted to go! The driver's attitude was "when they're ready, they'll let me know, in the meantime we'll just drive". That cultural focus on the journey rather than the destination is such a contrast to the Western obsession with goals, targets, and deadlines (or the behavioural contract (Sills, 2006) in TA). A dialogic therapeutic attitude is driving without knowing the destination. This is more in line with exploratory or growth and discovery contracts (Sills, 2006). By abdicating control of the direction of dialogue or its outcome, Spinelli (2015) suggests that, paradoxically, we both have greater ownership over that dialogue as a true expression of the different current worldviews we both hold. To have a dialogic attitude, therefore, we need to tolerate uncertainty. This is described by the phenomenologist, Hans-Georg Gadamer:

> the way one word follows another, with the conversation taking its own twists and reaching its own conclusion, may well be conducted in some way, but the partners conversing are far less the leaders than the led. No one knows in advance what will "come out" of such a conversation.
>
> (Gadamer, 2004, p. 383)

Process rather than content

Likewise, it is important that we concentrate on the *process* of the communication rather than get stuck on the *content*. In relationship therapy I often notice that getting bogged down with the content is a way of partners discounting what is really being said, believed, thought, and felt (the ulterior transactions (Berne, 1964)); the problem is often not really the way their partner stacks the dishwasher but the fact that they are feeling disrespected, unheard, or not understood. It is similar with the therapeutic or consultative dyad. We need to look deeper than the topic or content and reflect on and talk about the way that content is being discussed and expressed in the immediacy of the therapeutic encounter (Heidegger, 1927/2010).

Penny

Penny, a woman in her 70s who came to see me because of relational difficulties, spent a great deal of time in sessions pastiming (Berne, 1964) about her everyday experiences. It often felt more like a chat between friends than a therapy session. Yet I was aware that as we talked and laughed, I was growing fond of Penny and I felt like she was growing fond of me. "I know we're talking about shopping, but it feels like we're really connecting, Penny. Is it the same for you?" I asked her one day. Penny didn't answer, but nodded slightly, and I noticed her cheeks blush a little whilst she gave a coy smile. She then returned to talk about the shopping she was going to do after the session, but I felt there was a new, vital energy emerging between us. She mentioned she needed to buy ground cumin, and, in a playful self-disclosure, I commented that I had not been able to find any recently because of food shortages during the Covid-19 pandemic. At our next session, Penny shyly placed a pot of ground cumin on the table next to her. "I bought this for you, Rachel, to remind you of me". And then, more playfully, "don't say I never give you anything!". It emerged that Penny had visited several shops to find it, and the sense of intimacy and vitality was unmistakeable as I shared how touched I was at her thoughtfulness and we laughed together at the oddness of the gift. We talked about the illustration of the cumin for our relationship and Penny's worldview, and we played with the different meanings of spices for Penny. We enjoyed the links with spices being traditionally used for medicinal purposes and the evocation of the phrase, "the spice of life". Penny could see that her vitality was growing, her physis emerging, and her worldview shifting as she was moving further into intimate relating, which was bringing a welcome "spiciness" to her life. Touchingly, I later discovered that cumin was historically carried by a bride and groom and soldiers at war to symbolise love, faithfulness, and togetherness, something that our pastiming had brought to our relationship through relinquishing control of our dialogue and finding a route into intimacy and encounter.

Illustration

The cumin was an example of the empathic transaction "illustration" (Berne, 1966; Hargaden & Sills, 2002), or "metaphorical attunement" (Spinelli, 2015): the use of imagery, metaphor, stories, and dreams by the therapist or client to get to the heart of something that can be difficult to put into words. Clients' subtle and unthought through use of illustration can be a powerful way of opening up dialogue in the therapeutic encounter, offering a novel route into their non-conscious worldviews. I also encourage them to bring their dreams, symbolism, and illustration and will usually share the images, symbols, fantasies, or mental pictures that come to my mind as we are talking to see if it has significance for them. Occasionally, after reflection in supervision, I may also share a dream I have had about them, with the aim of helping my client make greater sense of their world. Vital to the existential approach is the bracketing of my own meaning, preferences, prejudices, biases, and interpretations so that we can focus on the client's experience, meaning, and processes.

Dreams

The existential perspective sees dreams (and daydreams or fantasies) as potent expressions of a person's lived reality and as equally valid as their waking-world (Boss, 1977). Spinelli (2015), drawing on Heidegger's (1927/2010) "Being-in-the-World", describes them as an expression of the concerns of our embodied experience through our own private language. Rather than interpreting the unconscious symbolism of the dream, therefore, the existential therapist will open up and explore connections between the dream-world and the waking world. This enables the client to make their own meaning, often linked to their presenting problem or recent therapeutic dialogues. As Cohn argues: "[t]hey are not puzzles to be solved but openings to be attended to" (Cohn, 1997, p. 84).

It is a deeply intimate and trusting gift for someone to share the illustration of a dream with us and it needs to be explored respectfully. Descriptive inquiry about all aspects of the dream (remembering not to prioritise one aspect over another) helps them to explore the thoughts, feelings, behaviours, objects, and memories in the dream, and anything which is evoked through the process of description. This can often reveal the person's being and worldview in direct, raw, and unguarded ways, bringing non-conscious views, values, beliefs, disturbances, tensions, and fears into awareness and enabling them to play creatively with alternatives. Whilst I was writing about self-disclosure, I had a dream that I was at a public swimming pool. I looked down and noticed with alarm that I was semi-naked and that my body was wasting away. I was particularly upset that my breasts were disappearing but at the same time was relieved that this made the exposure more bearable. When I discussed the dream with my supervisor the next day, it was not difficult to make the connection between my dream-world and waking world in terms of the felt exposure of self-disclosing in my writing. What her inquiry of my dream gave me was the opportunity to describe and voice my fears and vulnerabilities and to clarify my values and beliefs about writing in a way that was authentic to my self and my work. As she asked me about the significance for me of my breasts, I was struck by the association with both giving out to others ("feeding"), as well as my sexuality. We discussed my need to be replenished and resourced, particularly with the time and energy needed for creativity of expression in the writing process. We also talked about my worldview on gender and sexuality, the vulnerability of being a woman at times and how exposure is often different for women than men, and the injustice of a cultural scripting (Shivanath & Hiremath, 2003) that regularly places expectations on women to be attentive to others' needs at the expense of their own. What a fantastic and unexpected resource I gave myself through my dream, and how helpful to engage in dialogue about it with a trusted and present other to bring a black-and-white dream into vivid technicolour.

Descriptive investigation

Structured enquiry and specification

Freud used the analogy of "archaeological digs" (1937) to describe the analytic process, whereas Binswanger (1942) – one of the first psychiatrists to engage with existential analysis – described the existential investigative process as "anthropology". Rather than digging into their past to provide interpretations of their difficulties, our work is to explore and illuminate the differing cultures, beliefs, expressions, behaviour, interactions, and aspirations of this unique (whilst also universally similar) and unknown human being. The bedrock of the dialogic attitude and existential approach is a "strategic questioning" (Peavey, 1997) that Spinelli (2015) calls "structured investigation". It is the closest thing to technique in the existential approach and is a phenomenological or descriptive enquiry that we might think of as Berne's interrogation or Hargaden and Sills' empathic enquiry. It is about relinquishing any assumptions about the client's worldview or script and seeking to help them describe and understand it, rather than offering our own explanations or interpretations. Specification or clarification is an essential aspect of descriptive investigation, as it enables the therapist to check their understanding, communicate this understanding to the client, and importantly to help the client hear their own words and see more clearly, accurately, and truthfully their worldview so they are free to keep or challenge it as they see fit. Trainees (and some experienced practitioners) sometimes discount the enormous potential in strategic questioning, thinking of it simply as a necessary signpost on the route to the more significant destination of interpretation, crystallisation, and change. For the existentialist, however, change is significant but is not something to be aimed for. More important is the non-judgemental acceptance of the person who is present (rather than their past or future self) and thereby helping them describe their experiences, beliefs, and worldview. This, in itself, is enough to evoke change: "To describe is to change" (Spinelli, 2015, p. 108).

Sometimes, because of our inquiry, the description continues for the client between sessions as they mull things over. Questioning is powerful. I remember my teenage son telling me that he had upset his girlfriend by not buying her something for Valentine's Day. "I shouldn't have to show someone I love them on a particular day of the year," he grumbled. "How *do* you show people you love them at other times?" I asked (admittedly, not entirely without an ulterior motive for change!). He was taken aback, floundered for a moment, then said thoughtfully, with a little embarrassment, "I'm not sure that I do". I left it there, as the inquiry had clearly been confrontative to his worldview. A few days later, he presented me with a beautiful bouquet of flowers, our short dialogue and my enquiry enabling him to reflect for himself about how he wanted to relate to the people he loved.

Phenomenological inquiry

Edmund Husserl (1931/2012), the founder of phenomenology, developed guidance for structured inquiry (Ihde, 1986) in the form of three rules: the rule of epoché (bracketing); the rule of description; and the rule of horizontalisation (or equalisation). *Bracketing* is being alert to our biases, values, beliefs, and assumptions, acknowledging that we cannot eradicate them but intentionally suspending them so that we do not impose them on our client. With *description*, we move away from the therapist's theoretical diagnosis, explanations, analysis, and interpretations and instead help the client to delve deeper into describing their experiences in more detail. In this way, we help them discover themselves and their worldview.

Adebayo

Adebayo was in turmoil about the meaning of his life and work as he described selling a failing business that had been his life project. In contrast, his current work was now about earning money rather than providing meaning and purpose. I was totally engaged in helping him find new meaning in life, but at every turn of our conversation I felt like I wasn't understanding him and, however hard I tried, he was getting increasingly frustrated with me. Finally, I admitted defeat. "I'm just not getting you today, am I, Ade?" "No," he replied, "It feels like you've got pre-conceived ideas about what work means, and it's not the same as mine". As we talked more, we realised that I was trying to help him discover fresh meaning in his new work, whereas he was wanting to fundamentally shift his way of thinking about work as meaning-making and find greater purpose down other avenues. I had not bracketed sufficiently my own values and beliefs about work and meaning-making to be fully available to help Adebayo describe his struggle with his changing worldview.

Husserl's third rule, that of *horizontalisation*, states that there is no hierarchy with any of the presenting possibilities and descriptions, and that we need to see all of them with equal meaning or significance. When my client's description provides different possible exploratory routes, I invite them to decide on the priority of direction rather than me imposing my view. However, because of my own biases, history, personality, and worldview, it is very easy – almost inevitable – for us to give greater significance to one description over another, and we need to be alert to rectifying this when it happens.

Pete

Pete described a moving and frequently recurring dream he had experienced since childhood, in which a daisy was gradually being subsumed by a sea of mud. I was struck by the associations with daisies and love and connection, getting lost in reveries about singing a love song about daisies to my children when they were babies, and as a child making daisy chains to give to my friends, or picking petals off one by one to see whether a boy loved me ("he loves me, he loves me not, he loves me..."). I started making mental theoretical interpretations, wondering whether his dreams were about his unmet needs for love and connection after his abandonment by his mother at a young age. I shared some of my associations with Pete, expecting it to be revelatory to him, but he looked at me blankly; what was so exciting for me was not hitting the spot for Pete! I realised that I was not bracketing my experiences and was imposing my interpretations on to him. I acknowledged my mistake and turned back to structured inquiry:

Rachel: "What do daisies mean for *you*, Pete?"
Pete: "I don't know really, I guess that's me in my dream."
Rachel: "And what does it feel like to be that daisy?"
Pete: "Suffocating... I can't get away from the mud".
Rachel: (Pause). What does it feel like to be suffocated, to not be able to get away?"
Pete: (clutching his chest) "I can't breathe, I'm fighting and struggling to get some air but I'm not strong enough, it's overpowering me."
Rachel: "And how does it feel to be overpowered?"
Pete: (Silence, then quietly) "Terrifying".
Rachel: (Silence, then quietly, holding my chest) "Yes... Terrifying ... I can feel that terror".

I felt the terror rising up in my own chest as I entered Pete's existential terror with him. For Pete in this moment, the mud was the figural part of the dream, not the daisy. I had not practiced horizontalisation but had instead prioritised (wrongly) one aspect of his dream as more significant than another. As I enabled him to choose the direction of our dialogue rather than decide for him the hierarchy of each aspect of his dream description, Pete was able to make his own interpretations and describe and crystallise his existential terror.

Inclusion

For Clark (1991) and Hargaden & Sills (2002), empathy is the critical factor in the effectiveness of our enquiry and specification. For the existential psychotherapist and consultant, it is "inclusion" (Buber, 1923/1958): the ability to put oneself as fully as possible into the other's experience without judging, analysing, or interpreting, whilst also not losing oneself in the client and retaining a sense of one's separate, autonomous presence. Inclusion provides a safe environment for the client and communicates an understanding of their experience, thereby increasing their self-awareness.

Acceptance

An important aspect of inclusion is that we show our understanding and acceptance of what is being described, without approval or disapproval, even if we do not agree. We have some expertise obtained through our training and experience, and we might have some wisdom gained through life and work experience, but we are not "expert" at being human. It is arrogant to assume that we know best how a fellow unique human being is to be helped. I am not the surgeon who removes splinters or the magician who turns the frog back into the prince or princess, I am the fellow struggling human being who is prepared to put on their wellington boots and wade into the mud with my client, without pathologising them.

Confirmation

Through the therapist's acceptance of the other (albeit with challenge), the client is invited to accept themself as they are, and therein lies the great paradox of change as advocated by the person-centred and Gestalt approaches: "the curious paradox is that when I accept myself as I am, then I change" (Rogers, 1990, p. 19). True acceptance is about confirming the presence and the being of the other, which Buber (1923/1958) describes as "confirmation". This is different from Berne's (1966) confirmation which supports a successful confrontation, reinforcing what the client has said and helping the client to make a shift to take in reality. An existential perspective to confirmation is about meeting and choosing to recognise the other and their different perspective or worldview, not assuming we know what reality is. It is about recognising the subjectivity of the other, with an acceptance of where and who they are but additionally holding a hope for what they can become and their capacity to reach their potential. It is an acceptance that they are balancing the polarities of fear and growth (mud and daisies) and being committed to staying with and standing beside them in their otherness, whilst also encouraging and celebrating their movement into growth rather than staying stuck in fear. To do so, I, too, must be continuing to grow and be able to accept and tolerate my own uncertainty, insecurity, vulnerability, and discomfort, knowing and accepting the "mud" that terrifies me.

Presence

Holding and potency

My presence, not my theory or technique, is the most important thing I can offer my clients, supervisees, and students. It is my personal qualities and the quality of the immediacy of the therapeutic encounter that really makes a difference therapeutically, and experiencing my presence is one way that supervisees and students can learn how to bring their presence to their clients, and for clients to offer their presence to other relationships. This is partly (but not fully) accounted for in TA by the concepts of potency (Steiner, 1968), protection, permission (Steiner, 1966; Crossman, 1966), and holding (Hargaden & Sills, 2001, 2002). Hargaden and Sills refer to presence in their definition of their "holding" transaction: "The steady containing *presence* of a non-judgemental therapist who is perceived as having the potency to offer the protection and permission needed" (Hargaden & Sills, 2002, p. 127, my emphasis). Steiner also links potency with holding, describing it as the ability of the therapist to hold the client's despair in existential crisis: "Potency is …exemplified in protection by the willingness of the therapist temporarily to carry the burden of the patient's panic when in an existential vacuum" (Steiner, 1968, p. 63).

Confrontation of script and worldview

As well as holding and potency, presence involves confrontation. Berne described potency as "the power to confront" (Berne, 1972/1992, p. 375), but his view of confrontation is different from the existential perspective. For Berne and Hargaden and Sills, confrontation is about highlighting inconsistencies and challenging contaminated beliefs. However, this assumes that we have a judgement of what is or is not a contamination, and that our view is the correct one. In the existential approach confrontation is instead about offering a challenge to the client's worldview and thereby bringing into awareness their unconscious "dissociations and sedimentations" (Spinelli, 2015) so that the client can decide with greater clarity how they want to live.

This existential concept of sedimentation can be linked directly to the TA perspective of script, ego states, the contaminations of the Adult ego state, and the confusions of the Child ego state. Whilst transactional analysts may envision the unconscious, split-off, disowned, denied, or disavowed aspects of self and personal and family history in the depths and reaches of Child ego states, existentialists use the analogy of "sediments" on the river floor of life that give us a solid but false sense of identity and dam up our life (van Deurzen & Adams, 2016). Sedimentations defensively and ingeniously aim to maintain the safety and stability of our worldview, a direct parallel with TA's Parent and Child ego states that provide the security but rigidity of life script. Both are ways to describe what keeps us stuck or resistant to challenge at the cost of some aspect of our existence.

Much like the TA practitioner with contaminations and confusions, the existential practitioner aims to confront and bring these sedimentations and dissociations into awareness. However, for the existentialist, this is not because they judge their client's worldview as pathological (in the way that Berne describes script), but to help highlight existential tensions and to encourage them to consider whether they want to keep their worldview or look at other perspectives, beliefs, or views. Worldview from an existential perspective is more in line with Heiller and Sills' (2010) existential perspective on script as meaning-making, and the contemporary constructivist view of script as an ongoing life narrative that can be a constructive, dynamic, and creative way of helping people understand their life story and make sense of their existence (Cornell, 1988; English, 1988; Allen & Allen, 1997; Summers & Tudor, 2000). Confronting such a worldview is about being the antagonist to the other's life project (Sartre, 1943/1956), and it is through the therapist's authentic presence that they can be the most effective antagonist to the client's worldview and their ways of being-in-the-world. The felt sense of the authenticity of the therapist, however uncomfortable that may be, offers the client a protected space which enables them to gradually bring their authentic self into awareness and into the relationship. This gives potency to the relationship (Tudor & Summers, 2014), enabling the client to give themselves permission to challenge their worldview and crystallises their options for present and future relating and ways of being.

Games and existential impasses

It is through the microcosm of this therapeutic encounter that the macrocosm of the client's inter-relational possibilities and limitations outside the therapy room can be explored and expressed (Cohn, 1997; Spinelli, 2001). Transactional analysts may think of this in terms of games (Berne, 1964), interpersonal impasses (Cornell & Landaiche, 2006), interlocking rackets, or scripts (Holtby, 1979), interlocking relational impasses (Hemlin, 2012) or enactments (Cook, 2012; Shadbolt, 2012; Novak, 2015; Sills & Stuthridge, 2016). Relational transactional analysts attempt to work with enactments to bring the client's unconscious dynamics into awareness and, by repairing ruptures, provide a relational experience that is different from past relationships. Some of these theories unfortunately imply that one or both parties are relating pathologically, or that the client has more responsibility for these dynamics than the therapist. In contrast, Cornell & Landaiche (2006) describe interpersonal impasses in the therapeutic or consultative relationship arising because of the growing intimacy between them. The intimacy evokes both of their earliest unconscious relational patterns ("protocol" (Berne, 1961)), which is not necessarily pathological but creates an impasse between them, both because of their movement into health and their defences against the deepening affect and intimacy. This view has similarities with Spinelli's "embodied existential insecurities in relationship" (Spinelli, 2015, p. 68).

From an existential perspective, disturbances in the therapeutic or consultative relationship are not thought about as pathological or simply as relational patterns that are specific to these individuals and this particular dyad, but as unresolvable and inevitable universal conflicts, paradoxes, "existence tensions", and "existential polarities" (Wahl, 2003). These tensions are "intrinsic to human experience" (Wahl, 2003, p. 267) and underpin all human existence, and I therefore find it helpful to think of these as *"existential impasses"*. The presence of the practitioner can uncover existential impasses for the client because of their inevitably different worldview – their histories, personalities, beliefs, values, priorities, feeling responses, bodily experiences. Difficulties can emerge for the individual or in the dyad when we become polarised in one extreme of these polarities, stuck in a place of "either/or" rather than "both/and": life *or* death, power *or* powerlessness, work *or* play, acceptance *or* rejection, attachment *or* separation, avoidance *or* confrontation, control *or* letting go. It can be more productive to see each tension in terms of a continuum of "both/and": responsibility *and* freedom, conventionality *and* uniqueness, ritual *and* spontaneity, security *and* risk, conflict *and* harmony, belonging *and* isolation, intimacy *and* withdrawal, meaning *and* meaninglessness, love *and* hate, continuity *and* change. However, there is an inevitable tension and anxiety that comes with the freedom of the both/and rather than the rigidity and certainty of the either/or. Spinelli (2015) says that wherever we locate ourselves on each continuum will provoke tension because it means we have the anxiety of not being located at another point on the continuum. Existential impasses are thus an inevitable part of life and relationships; when we are faced with another person at a different point on the same continuum, we can experience increasing tension and anxiety because it holds up a mirror to our differences. This can be particularly acute in an intimate relationship when faced with existential tensions at the boundaries of the relationship (money, time, closeness/distance, differentiation of self/other, power/powerlessness).

A much-valued supervisee and I had a strong disagreement over changing our in-person meeting to a virtual session; I did not want to change, she felt I was being unfair and inflexible. When I explained my reasons but she continued to argue with me about it, I felt angry at my boundaries being disrespected. When I became angry with her, she felt hurt and misunderstood; when she became self-protective and told me she did not know if she wanted supervision with me anymore, I felt hurt. We can think of the dynamics between us as a game or enactment around power, authority, respect, rejection, or abandonment, and no doubt in that moment we each triggered for the other something of past relational patterns. However, what I think ultimately helped us both was not for one or both of us to be shoe-horned into changing our ways of relating, but in staying present with the ensuing uncomfortable and painful tussle. To acknowledge our differences and reach a greater understanding of ourselves and each other through confrontative dialogue. As both of us gradually accepted responsibility for our own worldviews and how they impacted the other, we were able to make meaning together, bring non-conscious aspects of our worldviews into awareness, and move from our entrenched or polarised "I–It" relating to more fluent "I–Thou" relating, without losing our own perspective. Stern describes it as a "shared meaning voyage" (Stern, 2004a, p. 172), and with meaning comes greater existential choice for present and future relating. Interestingly, neither of us fundamentally changed our positions. They were not right or wrong but were inevitable existential tensions around power/powerlessness, responsibility/freedom, control/letting go. What changed was that we both became less polarised through accepting the other's position and our differences, and embracing movement along the continuum of the polarities.

It can be helpful to think about existential impasses with any of the couple relationships we work with. It is a common cause of difficulties in relating and communication: one wants more intimacy, the other wants more time alone. One takes a great deal of responsibility, the other appreciates freedom. One likes to control, the other feels the need to let go. One plans meticulously, the other is more spontaneous. Our aim is not to "resolve" existential impasses, but to make meaning of our shared humanity and clarify where each of us is positioned on the continuums of life's paradoxes and polarities, and to explore and describe the resulting anxiety and the difficulties they have with tolerating the other's orientation. It is often the description in itself that leads to movement from the stuck place of either/or to the more fluid both/and: cooperation *and* competition. I am not talking about the compromise of merging into a dull middle ground, but about expanding possibilities and to "become able to accommodate greater contrast in self and others. The existential goal is to master the use of colour rather than settle for dull grey" (van Deurzen, 2012, p. 67).

The four inter-relational realms

As the therapeutic relationship deepens, trust and ease with immediacy grows, humour is employed and responded to in their discourse, and challenges are accepted and even initiated by the client, Spinelli (2015) suggests that existential work can shift from attunement to the client's worldview to exploration of the client and therapist's experience of being in relation with one another. He describes this as movement from the "I-focused" and "You-focused" inter-relational realms to the "We-focused" realm. This is similar to the intersubjectivity of co-creative TA's philosophy of "we-ness". Existentially, it is about engagement with our real and valid similarities, differences and "otherness", rather than pathologising our encounters as simply the client's transference.

It is through the challenging immediacy of our relating that we can illuminate and clarify the inter-relational existential issues that our client experiences in both the therapeutic relationship and in the wider world. Such immediacy of encounter can be "beguiling, uncanny, liberating, disturbing, intimate, desirable and undesirable both for and between the therapist and the client"

(Spinelli, 2015, p. 167). It can therefore be easy for therapists who have diffi-culty with the immediacy or intimacy of the We-focused realm to escape to the safety of theory, interpretation or the I-focused domain, disappearing behind the mask of the therapist role. But for the courageous practitioner, taking the risk to be vulnerable by disclosing something of themselves and their thoughts, feelings and experiences offers the potential for great therapeutic reward.

Self-disclosure

The potential rewards of this fifth and final existential transaction – therapist self-disclosure – are often sacrificed because of the significant risks associated with it to both client and therapist. I cannot do justice in a few paragraphs to the possibilities and perils of this inevitable, powerful, and sometimes contro-versial transaction, so have devoted the next chapter to its exploration. In it, I explore the different types of self-disclosure, the legacy of shame surrounding therapist disclosure, the risks to both client and therapist – and some of the mistakes I have made – and the importance of mitigating the risks by never los-ing sight of our role. But I also advocate for ethical risk-taking and experimen-tation. Having the courage to self-disclose – with appropriate ethical care – can lead to greater client empowerment; an increase in awareness, authenticity, and transparency; a sense of shared humanity and universality; the development of human care, mutuality, and intimacy; the integration of creative and destruc-tive behaviours, thoughts, and feelings; impasse clarification or resolution; and greater erotic vitality in life. I do not believe that we can help people become more fully and beautifully human if we do not share something of the reality of our humanity with them. Like my dream at the public swimming pool, we need to be open to the exposure of being metaphorically semi-naked if we are to work with authenticity. So, with curiosity and courage let's dive right in to the next chapter and explore the powerful, creative and contentious existential transaction that is self-disclosure.

Chapter 4

Self-disclosure

Going behind the mystical curtain of our role

The legacy of shame around self-disclosure

Self-disclosure is both inevitable and vital in a relational and existential psychotherapy. Yet it remains one of the most personal and contentious interventions in the psychotherapy field. By self-disclosure, I mean the many different ways the practitioner consciously, non-consciously, and unconsciously reveals something of themselves to their client, initiated by either the client or the therapist. I consider later the risks and benefits of self-disclosure in five different contexts: disclosure of the therapist's personal style and the workings of therapy (Yalom, 2002); disclosure of the therapist's personal life; disclosure of the therapist's countertransference; disclosure of the therapist's present reality; and disclosure of the therapist's humanity or "being". How much a therapist chooses to reveal of themselves in each of the different forms is a deeply personal decision, dependent on their personality, their personal philosophy, and their methodology of psychotherapy. Yet there is still a lingering cultural scripting in the psychotherapy field that leaves many therapists who disclose their real selves feeling "transgressive" and with a sense of shame. "I have found my own therapist's disclosures of her humanity really helpful to lessen my shame about my imperfections," said one of my supervisees, "yet I cannot get over the shame I feel when I disclose to my own clients. I feel like I'm doing something really wrong as a therapist".

Whilst there is now a wide spectrum of contemporary perspectives on self-disclosure in transactional analysis (TA) and existential psychotherapy, I think this sense of transgressive shame goes back to the legacy of psychoanalysis, where the analyst was expected to be the blank screen on to which the client projected their unconscious material. Any type of self-disclosure was therefore considered largely inappropriate. With TA originating from Berne's psychoanalytic history, it is no wonder that there are still remnants of shame around the concept and practice. And, of course, the cultural shame may tap into the therapist's (or Eric Berne's) own personal shame around intimacy or exposing their vulnerabilities. In the existential field, many phenomenologists also consider that Husserl's (1931/2012) concept of "bracketing" or epoché

DOI: 10.4324/9781003475217-6

precludes self-disclosure, believing that it is the therapist's job to enter the client's lived experience, not for the client to enter theirs. But bracketing does not mean excluding. Husserl, the founder of phenomenology, was a mathematician and the brackets or parentheses in a mathematical equation show the order of operations: the content of the brackets must be worked out first before bringing it into the rest of the equation. In existential psychotherapy, bracketing therefore means to first stop and consider our own perspectives, biases, and experiences so that we do not unintentionally impose them on our client.

Self-disclosure is risky and I agree with Hargaden and Sills that it is "so important yet potentially so open to misuse" (Hargaden & Sills, 2002, p. 129). Bracketing and reflexivity keeps us alert to this. Yet I suggest in this chapter that enabling our clients to enter our lived reality – as well as us entering theirs – can sometimes be transformational. Appropriate acknowledgement of our shared but unique and different humanity can offer our clients a deeper quality of relating that may help them become more aware of their own lived reality, make greater sense of their existence, appreciate the universalities and diversity of the human experience of life and relating, and help them move into greater authenticity and intimate relational encounter.

The risk of self-disclosure: never lose sight of your role

Risks to the client

Self-disclosure is risky to our clients because of the asymmetry of power in the therapeutic relationship. There is *always* an ethical dilemma associated with a disclosure because of the inevitable uncertainty about the outcome. Yet we can also never know what the consequences of our non-disclosure will be (Cornell, 2014). Even experienced, self-aware practitioners can easily eclipse the client through their self-disclosures, foreclosing on the client's process, or making it more about the therapist and their narcissistic needs. It can leave the client feeling confused, intruded upon, or burdened, unable to manage the therapist's humanity or vulnerability. It can invite an idealisation or denigration of the therapist, be about relieving the therapist's discomfort from holding something, or can implicitly encourage the client to adapt to the therapist (or be interpreted in this way). Whilst all practitioners need ongoing supervision around their self-disclosure, beginning therapists particularly need supervisory assistance to learn to contain their own process whilst developing their capacity for immediacy. Whatever their experience, my advice to supervisees is to remember the asymmetry of the relationship and never lose sight of their role as therapist.

Risks to the practitioner

The intimacy and vulnerability of self-disclosure also makes it risky for the therapist or consultant. We leave ourselves open to being hurt by our client's responses, and it has the potential to resurface unprocessed and overwhelming feelings, wounds, or memories. The intimacy of self-disclosure makes the emergence of sexual, romantic, or loving feelings for both client and therapist more likely, which, as long as it is not acted out inappropriately, is clearly not transgressive but can feel unmanageable and painful for both. The threat of getting the self-disclosure wrong can also leave therapists fearing facing complaints and ethics committees. The most pain and vulnerability I have experienced in my work as a therapist, supervisor, and teacher has been because of my self-disclosures, examples of which I offer later. The associated uncomfortable and humbling memories and residual shame make me non-judgemental of any practitioner who chooses to be cautious in this area.

Ethical risk-taking and ethical experimentation

But for a vital and enlivening psychotherapy we must also be prepared to take ethical risks. We cannot avoid pain, suffering, and uncertainty in life, relationships, or therapy, and more often than not my disclosures that have resulted in pain have also led to the greatest rewards of growth, learning, and transformation –for me as well as my clients. Like mountaineering, you cannot reap the rewards of the summits if you do not accept the risks. I would rather risk bearing the scars of a loving, challenging, vulnerable, intimate, and authentic relationship than to remain remote and isolated behind the impregnable walls of self-protection. But like the mountaineer, I advocate a measured rather than reckless risk in ethically thought-through self-disclosure. Such risk-taking brings colour and vitality into life and relationships, and I think it is our ethical responsibility to keep taking risks with experimentation so that we do not stagnate. How else are we to keep growing, develop therapeutic thinking and ideas, and discover more about ourselves and humanity? Whilst R.D. Laing's sometimes dubious boundaries brought criticism from many, I am inspired by his courageous and revolutionary approach that challenged the status quo of detached and pathologising psychiatry and psychotherapy. We need to overcome our fear of making mistakes and accept that they are inevitable, necessary, and potentially rewarding if we devote ourselves to helping both client and therapist learn and grow through them (Cook, 2012).

Mitigating the risks

Disciplined spontaneity

Of course, we need to do what we can to mitigate the risks, thinking ethically and caring deeply about our clients and ourselves. Eusden's (2023) "high-dare-high-care" ethical compass suggests that the greater the risk, the more ethical care needed. With self-disclosure, this means increasing amounts of attentive and challenging supervision, commitment to reflexivity, earning the right in relationship to self-disclose, privileging the client's needs over our own, and respecting their prerogative to decide that they do not want our disclosure. We also need to remember that self-disclosure will be different for each unique person and at various stages of their therapeutic journey. It is often too difficult for a new client to tolerate in the beginning phases of their therapy, or for the therapist to manage in the early stages of their career. Disclosures are often more effective and appropriate with longer-term clients, supervisees, and students where there is greater mutuality. But even then, we must avoid overshadowing, intruding, or imposing by never losing sight of our role.

Most important is a commitment to disciplined reflexivity – before, during, and after disclosure – through honest, challenging, and forthright supervision and personal therapy, a commitment to self-reflection and ongoing learning, and the cultivation of the ability to listen and respond to embodied intuition. Whilst disclosure might not be immediate (and may take months or even years until the time feels right), such discipline enables us to offer courageous disclosures with tentativeness, curiosity, and humility in the spontaneity of the present moment. Barsness and Strawn (2018) describe this as "disciplined spontaneity". This requires the courage and non-defensiveness to be able to hold the tension, uncertainty, and risk of disclosure. One of my supervisees found that self-disclosure of his experience in relationships was usually manageable with individuals but that two or more people in couples or groups made self-disclosure too anxiety provoking, risking his withdrawal or defensive attack. He rightly decided to hold back on disclosing until he felt less threatened:

> To speak courageously, the analyst must have a healthy respect for anxiety and tension without feeling threatened, hold direct requests for acknowledgement non-defensively and with curiosity, value his/her words as a means for exploration rather than as correctness, and finally, follow the patient's response.
>
> (Barsness & Strawn, 2018, p. 198)

Dialogue around self-disclosure

As far as possible we need to discover whether our client would find it beneficial for us to disclose and ask their permission in a moment-by-moment contract (Sills, 2006). For example, "Would you like to hear how I feel about that?"; "Are you up for hearing my responses to what you just said?"; "Would it be helpful for you to hear a bit about my experience with that?". We also need to keep a reflexive stance to monitor ourselves and our client's response in the immediacy of our disclosure, and to enquire of our client afterwards what the impact of the disclosure was for them. A good reflective exercise with any explicit disclosure is to ask ourselves "what, why, how, when?": *what* are we going to disclose, *why* do we think this will be beneficial for our client, *how* will we do it, and *when* will be an appropriate time? If I feel an urgency to disclose, I usually do not, but give myself more time to reflect on the reasons for the insistence. It can often be about my own desire for intimacy, empathy, soothing, twinning, and/or an invitation into sameness, which may foreclose on necessary disturbance.

When faced with direct questions about my personal life or responses I often give myself contemplation time, holding curiosity about the reasoning behind the question and reflecting on whether or not I want to disclose. Before answering, I may ask how they would feel to hear various responses to their question, but I usually prefer not to impose my power by being avoidant or withholding in insisting we first explore the reasons for their question. But I will always investigate what it was like for them to ask the question and how they are responding to our dialogue and my disclosure or non-disclosure. Any subsequent emergence of existential feelings and experiences of anger, frustration, embarrassment, shame, dislike, hate, withdrawal, envy, or rejection can provide fruitful routes into exploring and clarifying their ways of relating. If I don't want to self-disclose about my personal life I may disclose about my response to the question, such as, "I'm feeling uncertain about how to answer that question and would like some time to think about it." Or, "I'm not sure I want to answer that question immediately because I'm finding myself feeling defensive. Can we talk about that?" or even, "Your question makes me feel uncomfortable, like I'm being intruded upon in some way. Is that what you intended?" Ultimately, with the risk of any disclosure we must inquire of ourselves whether the potential rewards for the client are worth the risk to both client and practitioner. Will my disclosure "serve to further clarify the inter-relation between the client's presenting issues and his or her worldview" (Spinelli, 2015, p. 192), and, "do I think this will help my client to better understand themselves and their life?" (van Deurzen & Adams, 2016, p. 78).

The rewards of self-disclosure

The decision to self-disclose is deeply personal and will vary from practitioner to practitioner, from client to client, and from session to session. We constantly balance the existential tension of risk and reward, privacy and transparency, and our professional role and our humanity. To find our personal equilibrium we need to understand our chosen philosophy of psychotherapy and, more specifically, that of self-disclosure. My philosophy of authenticity and transparency means that I am committed to bringing my humanity into the therapeutic, supervisory, and educational encounter. This does not always require self-disclosure of my personal life, but I will no doubt share my humanity and disclose more broadly and frequently than some. The clinical examples in this chapter describe the outcomes of some of these disclosures. Occasionally they have been unhelpful, sometimes indifferent, and often rewarding. I now turn to look at the five different types of self-disclosure and examine the significant potential for existential rewards in the following ways:

1 Greater client empowerment
2 Increase in awareness, authenticity and transparency
3 A sense of shared humanity and universality
4 Development of care, mutuality and intimacy
5 Integration of creative and destructive behaviours, thoughts and feelings
6 Impasse clarification or resolution
7 Greater erotic vitality in life

Disclosure of the workings of therapy

One of the least contentious forms of self-disclosure – but not necessarily the most widely practiced – involves the therapist disclosing at the start of therapy how they work and what the client can realistically expect from therapy or consultation. For transactional analysts, this is an important aspect of open communication: bilateral contracting, making overt any unhelpful psychological contracts (Berne, 1961), and ensuring client empowerment. This is clearly harder for the beginning practitioner (who is not yet clear about their personal style), and there is a risk we might foreclose on therapeutic possibilities if we become too rigid. Disclosing how we are seeing the work evolving can be important when working existentially to establish that we are alongside our client rather than ahead of them in planning their treatment.

What is sometimes not considered or enquired about is what the client would like from their therapist, supervisor, consultant, or teacher. Are they hoping for a more supportive or challenging relationship? What would help them learn? What is their "job description" for the role they are hiring me for? Such enquiry offers, from the beginning of therapy, a dialogic attitude and possibilities for immediacy in the therapeutic encounter. It also sometimes highlights that we are not in fact a good match. One of my supervisees and I kept getting entangled in difficult dynamics until I realised that I had not asked her how she wanted me to be as a supervisor. When I did, I realised that what she wanted would not enable me to be authentic. "I cannot be someone I'm not", was my response. Our further explorations uncovered a mutual psychological contract where we *both* needed or wanted the other to be something or someone we were not. We parted ways respectfully, both of us having learned from the immediacy of our disclosures. Of course, this job description will evolve as they do and as the therapy or learning environment progresses. In a twist of fate, some years later I became her tutor. Having both changed and developed in the intervening years, we were now able to meet each other more fully and productively in our differences as the people we authentically were, not what we needed or thought the other to be.

Disclosure of the practitioner's personal life

Generally viewed with significantly more caution in TA, and in psychotherapy in general, is explicit disclosure of the therapist's personal life (Clarkson, 1992; Hargaden & Sills, 2002; Little, 2011, Novak, 2016). It is easy to forget that we often implicitly disclose something of our personal life (particularly when working from home) through the area in which we live or work, our therapy room, our books, the cats that greet them, the children's toys in the garden, our clothing, the words we choose, our voice and accent, our colour, our bodily expression. I had not considered the communication of my privilege through the paintings in my therapy room until one of my clients suggested that they spoke of my higher social class. It was a humbling lesson to me about how our privilege, power, and intersectional identity (Crenshaw, 1989) – and our experiences of oppression – oozes out of every pore. Sometimes their interpretation is inaccurate. One of my clients fantasised that a different car in my driveway meant that someone else in my life would mean less of my investment in her. Once we had explored the fantasy, disclosure of the reality (that it was my plumber's car!) helped throw light on her chasm between fantasy and actuality that was keeping her stuck in the existential polarities of envy, competition, and hostility.

To feel empathy for another human being we draw on our own life experiences, and our intuitive clients often speak of "knowing" that we have been through something similar to them. Spinelli (2015) describes this as "covert" disclosure. We do not need to bare all to be authentic, and we must respect our clients' "right not to know" more than is useful for them about our private lives (Oates & Kuchuck, 2016). Sometimes it is a very long time, if at all, before a traumatised or disturbed client is able to see the humanity of the therapist or move out of objectifying transferential dynamics. In these instances, it is entirely appropriate for us to focus instead on entering their reality rather than trying to impose ours onto them. But openness, honesty, and transparency – and making explicit the implicit – can often inspire trust, bring a sense of relief or identification with a fellow human being, and help them make meaning of their own experiences.

When self-disclosure goes wrong

It does not always go to plan. I have sometimes disclosed too much or too soon for my clients, sought differentiation when they have still needed twinship, or consciously or non-consciously invited sameness when they have therapeutically required differentiation. There have been instances when my clients have left therapy because they have felt adrift at the loss of containment or the cutting through of the idealisation, felt intruded upon by the self-disclosure, or have swiftly moved from idolisation to denigration of me or the therapy.

Irena

I think, with a touch of shame and regret, of my client, Irena, who left in a rage, never to return, after I disclosed a recent bereavement. "Don't bring your grief here," was her angry response, "this is not about you". My intention was to help her identify with both my humanity and her own sequestered grief, to enable a move from objectification into intersubjectivity. But in sharing my vulnerability, I think that I touched too early on her own vulnerability and shame-evoking private parts of self that she was not yet ready to open up to – her hidden core self that Winnicott (1963) describes as the "isolate". For deeply traumatised people, this is the part of self that, whilst longing to be seen, is more terrified of being found. In angrily ending therapy, Irena kept her "isolate" and shame safely hidden, and left me with a cocktail of shame, fear, anger, and sadness that probably belonged to both of us. Through this humbling and painful experience, I learnt more about my own potential for intrusion, the risk for me in being wounded because of my self-disclosure, and the importance of respecting my clients' right to distance and privacy.

Destruction and creation

Yet, I also don't want experiences such as this to make me risk-averse. However difficult or painful our struggle, if both are willing to dialogue and engage with our differences, it is possible to move towards mutual recognition (Benjamin, 1990) and find meaning and transformation in the rupture that self-disclosure has caused.

Thomas

This was demonstrated with my client, Thomas, who was persistently asking me playfully and flirtatiously to disclose whether I was married. Sensing his seduction, and still feeling vulnerable after my own painful divorce, I decided not to self-disclose my personal life but disclosed instead my feelings of being seduced. Over several years, our engaging tussle around seductiveness developed into what seemed like greater intimacy and more respectful curiosity about my marital status. In an attempt at deepening our intimacy further, I told him I was divorced.

He was dumbfounded. "But how can you be a therapist and not even make your own relationships work? What's wrong with you?" he threw at me with an unvetted and hurtful outrage. I felt my cheeks flush and a sense of failure and shame overwhelm me, both because of my decision to disclose that had caused such a rupture, as well as the remnants of shame and vulnerability about my relational breakdown. Our masks had been stripped away. I fumbled through the rest of the session in a desperate attempt to hold on to my dignity and over several months (and with my therapist and supervisors alongside me) we explored my therapeutic mistake and the alienation of our rupture. I disclosed the emotional impact he had on me, Thomas described his discombobulation at seeing me as vulnerable and imperfect, and we both admitted the judgement we held towards each other. We investigated his beliefs about marriage, divorce, power, and women, and how these presented in our relating, as well as the erotic connection between us. He revealed his fantasy that because I was divorced, I was now "available", and this terrified him: his seductiveness was a mask that was only manageable when the other was at a safe distance, and the shifting of the boundaries around disclosure felt too intimate.

I am not sure I would have chosen the hurt of that experience with Thomas, but I am ultimately glad to have had the encounter. Through meeting each other without masks, we experienced each other's failings, imperfections, shame, judgements, vulnerabilities, anxieties, and desires, and Thomas became much more aware of his worldview and ways of relating. We both experimented with deeper levels of intimacy and I developed in accepting and revealing my vulnerability in service of the relationship: "The analyst's role is not defined by invulnerability, in other words, but by a special (though inconsistent) willingness, and a practiced (though imperfect) capacity to accept and deal with her vulnerability" (Stern, 2004a, p. 216). Many would consider it "rupture and repair" but I think "destruction and creation" is more apt. Rollo May (1969) describes the "Daimonic" as a universal aspect of human existence that is the expression of both creative and destructive behaviours, thoughts and feelings. Through my self-disclosure, Thomas and I had channeled the "destructive" and thereby enabled the potentiality of the "creative": our old relationship had been destroyed and we had worked together to create a new one on the old foundations.

Developing care, mutuality, and intimacy

Self-disclosure of our private lives does not always lead to such enactments, as I show with my long-standing client, Freja.

Freja

Disclosing my bereavement to Freja proved to be profoundly connecting, confronting of her existential tensions and worldview, and enabled greater mutuality in relationship. In the week after my friend died, Freja noticed that I was a little subdued and asked whether I was okay. Wanting to affirm her intuition, I disclosed my bereavement, reassuring her that I was indeed okay but that she was probably picking up my underlying sadness at my loss. I was deeply touched by the genuine empathy and concern she showed me. She had known significant bereavement in her life and was able to communicate her presence and care by gently and respectfully asking me questions about my friend. What a role reversal! Yet I never forgot that I was therapist, nor the therapeutic reasons for my disclosure. When I enquired about what this had been like for her, Freja reported that changing roles – whilst knowing that I was still holding my position as therapist – provided her with a sense of kinship, a mutuality between us, and a feeling of significance and confidence in being able to express her care for me. She said that my disclosure also normalised her experiences of bereavement and grief, which enabled her to address at greater depth existential themes of death, loss, anxiety, injustice, uncertainty, friendship, love, and intimacy. For Freja, the rewards of my self-disclosure were well worth the risk.

Impasse resolution

Sometimes it can be helpful for us to initiate a personal self-disclosure, particularly when we are facing an interpersonal impasse (Cornell & Landaiche, 2006; Little, 2011).

Aisha and Rebecca

Aisha, an experienced supervisee, and her client, Rebecca, were stuck. Aisha had attempted but failed to help clarify Rebecca's seeming intrapsychic impasse (Goulding & Goulding, 1978; Mellor, 1980) around wanting to withdraw from a religious "cult". Feeling misunderstood because of their different histories, Rebecca had become increasingly withdrawn. Aisha invited exploration into what was happening between them, disclosing to Rebecca her feelings of being stuck, but this served simply to increase their shared frustration and sense of alienation. "The thing is", Aisha said to me, "I *won't* understand her, because I just don't have the same religious beliefs as her". "Does she know that?", I enquired. "No, she's never asked". I wondered about her client's lack of curiosity and my supervisee's unusual lack of transparency, observing that their difference seemed to be frightening them both, shutting down the mutual investigation. "What would it be like to ask her if she wants to know anything about your beliefs?", I enquired. "I can't possibly do that!", she exclaimed, looking startled and anxious. "It might be too much for her and make her leave". "Yes, it might, that's certainly a risk", I replied, "but at least it will open up the conversation about your differences and you'll both me more open to discovering truth".

Aisha and I explored together her own fears around difference and abandonment, and in our next supervision session she reported that she had indeed asked Rebecca if there was anything she wanted to know about her religious beliefs. "I almost don't think it mattered what my answer was", Aisha told me, "It was just important to her that I was open and willing to acknowledge that I could not truly understand her situation". Facing their existential impasses around connection and isolation relieved the tension of the interpersonal and intrapsychic impasses, enabling their further exploration around belonging, freedom, and individuation.

The stifling of Rebecca and Aisha's curiosity through fear had led to a deadening of their erotic relating, the life force of physis, which Mann describes as "the very creative stuff of life" (Mann, 1997, p. 4). Without creativity, impasses solidify. I talk about self-disclosure around the erotic in Chapter 13, but in general we need to differentiate between the curiosity that is intrusive, destructive, and hostile (an eroticised distancing, as it was initially with Thomas), and an erotically enlivening "philosophical wonder" (Heidegger, 1927/2010). I do not want to shut down the latter, as this can suggest that there is something in their erotic vitality of which to be ashamed. Instead, meeting their creative curiosity about our lives with appropriate self-disclosure can bring passion and an erotic life-breath into the therapeutic encounter and into the lives of our clients.

Disclosure of the therapist's countertransference

A different form of self-disclosure became popularised in TA with the advent of the relational approach (Cornell & Hargaden, 2019; Fowlie & Sills, 2011; Hargaden & Sills, 2001, 2002), inspired by the work of American relational psychoanalysts (Aron, 1996; Bollas, 1988; Maroda, 1999; Mitchell, 1988). Rather than disclosing aspects of their personal life, the focus is on the therapist's "use of self" and judicious self-disclosure of the therapist's countertransference. The therapist's countertransference is considered to be the means by which they can hear the unconscious communication of the client's internal distress and relational dynamics. Whilst regrettably not including self-disclosure as one of their empathic transactions (arguing that any of the empathic transactions could involve self-disclosure), Hargaden and Sills described it as an additional operation that may help to bring unconscious relational dynamics into awareness and communicate to the client "a form of empathic understanding of the original protocol" (Hargaden & Sills, 2002, p. 130). When client and therapist recruit each other into defensive games and enactments, self-disclosure offers potential links between the therapeutic relational dynamics and those of their childhood, as well as providing a more positive relational experience as ruptures are worked through and hopefully repaired (Cook, 2012; Novak, 2015; Shadbolt, 2012; Sills & Stuthridge, 2016). Gabbard and Wilkinson describe such self-disclosure of our countertransference as a "clinical honesty", which involves informing the patient of the "interpersonal and intrapsychic use that the patient is making of the therapist" (Gabbard & Wilkinson, 1994, p. 143).

What is missing is the acknowledgement that the therapist will inevitably also be transferring their internal dynamics on to the client. If we simply focus on self-disclosing our countertransference in a way that interprets our client's "pathology", we position ourselves as the expert and discount our role in the co-transference. This is counter to the existential-phenomenological principle of meaning-making through descriptive investigation and a mutuality of dialogue. There is also a tendency to hold back on disclosing countertransference, but to use it silently to enable the client to make use of the therapist through the transferential dynamics. Whilst I believe that conscious, non-conscious, unconscious, and transferential dynamics are ever-present and inevitable (and their exploration is helpful), I am not of the opinion that withholding disclosure to deliberately encourage the deepening of the transference-countertransference relationship (Little, 2011) is always a kind, mutual, or ultimately productive method or methodology. I think such an approach may evoke a greater power differential and I prefer an existential stance that gradually (over months or years) invites each other out of transferential relating in order that we are able to recognise and understand our own and each other's humanity.

Disclosure of the therapist's present reality

Some authors in TA, drawing on Gestalt and Person-centred psychotherapy, have moved away from thinking about the therapeutic relationship as a transferential relationship and prefer to work solely with present-centred relating and a position of health rather than pathology (Tudor & Summers, 2014). Self-disclosure is therefore not about using countertransference as a means to help understand the client's historical "pathology" but about how they are experiencing the other and the therapeutic relationship in the here-and-now, present-centred moment of relating. In this way they use self-disclosure of the workings of the therapeutic relationship as a vehicle for exploration, change and growth, and the opportunity for different ways of relating. Widdowson's (2008) metacommunicative transactions provide a method for this form of disclosure.

I believe that it is never completely possible to differentiate between unconscious transferential/countertransferential relating ("what is mine, theirs or both") and what is here-and-now, conscious, non-transferential Adult relating. We can never know for sure which ego state we are coming from; more than that, there will inevitably be a mix of ego states at any one time. Our relating will always be a swirling blend of co-transferential and non-transferential relating: conscious, non-conscious and unconscious feelings, urges, thoughts, felt wisdom, fantasies, embedded memories, and bodily experiences; and phenomenally fast, complex, and often imperceptible shifts between ego states. However slight, our earliest imprints of relationship from our archaic past (our unconscious and embodied "protocol" (Berne, 1961)) will be informing how we relate to others today. Sometimes it will be a whisper of an embedded memory in response to a person's smile or passing touch, at other times a pang of longing when we receive love or attention that we previously lacked – or once had but have now lost – or a regression when someone's anger takes us back to our parent's uncontrollable wrath. We will also always relate unconsciously from a position of health as well as defensiveness: there will be repression, dissociation, denial, or disavowal, but also the health and vitality of our unconscious spirituality, sexuality, meaning-making, intelligence, wisdom, and values. In short, our unconscious – most of which will never become fully conscious – is part of our truth and our reality, our vital essence, our fundamental being. Self-disclosure of our responses can therefore never be considered as *either* disclosure of my countertransference *or* disclosure of my present-centred relating. I think it is always both. I therefore prefer to consider self-disclosure as disclosure of my present reality – which may or may not be different from my client's present reality. For both of us, our present reality is shaped by the other in this moment, as well as by all the imprints of both of our other historical relationships and life experiences. Self-disclosing our present reality with humility and awareness can therefore normalise their human struggle and experience, but also confront their worldview by offering a different perspective. In doing so, we may also uncover for deeper exploration the existential relational impasses and polarised positions with which we both may be grappling.

Yonita

An erotic, powerful, and passionate energy emerged when I felt betrayed by Yonita, a long-term client with whom I had been engaging in steady but unexciting work. I experienced a raw, embodied, and annihilating rage when she told me in passing that she had been seeing an old therapist at the same time as working with me. Much as I value immediacy, I knew my anger was disproportionate, and risked damaging our relationship if I spoke without enough Adult reflexivity present. As Hargaden and Sills warn, "Therapists' self-disclosure should always be "Adult ego state reporting on Child" rather than unmitigated Child" (Hargaden & Sills, 2002, p. 130). Yet I value honesty in the moment, so I disclosed my shock. "You seem angry," she responded. She is intuitive and I don't hide my emotions particularly well! I paused to reflect before affirming her intuition. "I am. I'm angry, upset and confused and I think I need some time to reflect on my response before we talk about it some more". We spent the remainder of the session in uncomfortable, honest, angry silence, which communicated more about our impasse than words ever could. As van Deurzen suggests, sometimes "keeping silent can be the most powerful way of having discourse" (van Deurzen 2010, p. 63).

In supervision and personal therapy, we contemplated the conscious, non-conscious, and unconscious dynamics between me and Yonita. Yes, my present reality was that I was appropriately angry at her disloyalty and lack of transparency, but I also had a complex history with betrayal and abandonment that was woven throughout my life. My present reality was therefore perhaps a melding of a here-and-now response to the current situation, a proactive countertransferential reaction to my own conscious and unconscious vulnerabilities that Yonita's relational decisions touched on, and perhaps a reactive countertransferential projective identification with some of Yonita's split-off rage. We were also potentially encountering an existential relational impasse: her need for withdrawal and my need for intimacy that was being played out in a tension between intrusion and abandonment. Not because of our "pathology", but because we had different personalities, histories, and protocols that were coming up against each other. This was not something to be resolved but was something universally human – whilst also unique to our relationship – that needed to be communicated about with a mutual empathy so that we could understand the other and discover how we both impacted each other.

Making sense in supervision of relational possibilities and my own present reality, without judgement or pathologising, enabled me to return to Yonita with greater curiosity and a desire to understand her, whilst not discounting my felt sense of betrayal. Without disclosing the specifics of my history, I gradually disclosed to Yonita my authentic anger and hurt, my fear that our relationship had been at risk, and my acknowledgement that she had touched some vulnerabilities for me because of my history and personhood. "Thank you for being honest with me, and thank you for protecting our relationship", she acknowledged sincerely and with relief. "It helps me to trust you." Our genuineness and transparency with our clients about our multi-layered process – without ever losing sight of the responsibility of our role – can bring a human touch to therapy that has the potential to reduce shame, build trust and intimacy, model a way of being, and lead to the client's greater acceptance of themselves and the challenges of life and relating. For Yonita, my disclosure enabled her to risk describing her anger and disappointment with me and our relationship. She told me about wanting more focus on the body from me, which her previous therapist offered, whilst also speaking of her fear of our emotional closeness: seeing both of us had helped to dilute the intensity of relating with me. Her visits to her previous therapist seemed to be a communication of both an erotic striving for growth and vitality, but also a retreat from erotic intimacy. And in highlighting, through our interpersonal impasse, my unconscious avoidance of the body, she offered me a much-appreciated challenge to my own embodied intrapsychic impasses that mirrored hers. Our mutual disclosures were not necessarily neatly resolving and ironing out our intrapsychic and interpersonal conflicts and impasses (although some revelation and relief from the tension was gained for both of us). But they were generating awareness and disturbance that moved us towards greater mutual understanding of our erotic and existential impasses around closeness, isolation, withdrawal, and intimacy.

Disclosure of the therapist's humanity or "being"

The real relationship in TA

In TA this shared humanity is described by Judy Barr as the "core relation-ship": "the relationship the client, as the person he or she really is in the here-and-now, has with the therapist, as the person the therapist really is in the present" (Barr, 1987, p. 137). Petruska Clarkson further suggests that "true psychotherapy only happens when therapist and patient find the person behind each other's defences". She defines the "real" or "I–You" therapeutic relation-ship as one "between *person-and-person* in the existential dilemma where both stand in a kind of mutuality to each other" (Clarkson, 1992, pp. 303–4). This is later echoed by Heiller and Sills who believe that "a mutual owning of the painful truths of life's journey can lie at the heart of the truly therapeutic rela-tionship" (Heiller & Sills, 2010, p. 263).

Sharing the existential dilemmas of humanity

Existentially, when we disclose that we do not have the answers to our client's difficulties, that we are stuck in the work, or that we have been hurt by our cli-ent, we illustrate that we all struggle with similar challenges in the face of the "impossible dilemmas of being human" (Spinelli, 2001, p. 168). Being coura-geously and humbly open with ourselves and our clients, supervisees, and stu-dents about our thoughts, feelings, sensations, intuitions, and the existential realities of life, models that we are truly accepting our individuality and that we, too, are always a process of "becoming" (Heidegger, 1927/2010) rather than seeing our self as a finished product. When we disclose the fullness of our humanity or our "being" – in words or an unspoken bodily or silent communi-cation – we can be credible and inspiring mentors to our clients (van Deurzen, 2015). We show that we are not so different from our client, that we are all human, and that it is possible to manage the universal difficulties and suffering of life (Yalom's (1985) "universality"). In seeing us as being human – and sur-viving – they can dare to search out the hidden recesses of their own humanity.

This disclosure of our humanity can also help them psychologically and spiritually. Maroda argues more generally for the therapist's willingness to be emotionally open: "It is the therapist's willingness to be forthcoming and to show emotion that is *curative* and stimulates emotional honesty" (Maroda, 1999, p. 103, original emphasis). Aron (1996) says that knowing something of the interior lives of their analysts also enables the development of the capacity to think psychologically. This can be particularly helpful for neurodivergent or traumatised people who have difficulties self-regulating or processing social cues, or who have more negative expectations and fantasies in relationship. R.D. Laing's (1960) existential-phenomenological approach with many deeply disturbed individuals was to be himself without masks, which, according to his clients, provided a "striking and genuine honesty" (Semyon, quoted in Mullan, 1997) that inspired a route into dialogue and encounter. This transparency and ability to experience the lived reality of the other can generate meaning and open up our clients to their spiritual dimension of existence, where "we no longer see ourselves as the centre of the universe but as part of a greater complexity to which we belong and owe our lives" (van Deurzen & Adams, 2016, p. 42). With a mutual transparency, we are more able to let the world in, be connected to it, and see all parts of life as connected and equally significant. We can find meaning in life and our own unique contribution to the world: "we have to aspire to be as transparent and open as possible so that 'light', existence, can shine in. When this happens, the person can simultaneously and reciprocally be lit up and light up the world" (van Deurzen & Adams, 2016, p. 42).

The need for privacy and "relational rest"

Whilst I am a great advocate for disclosure of my humanity, I also appreciate my need for privacy, reflection, contemplation, and the liminal space of "relational rest" (Corbett, 2014). Yonita taught me a great deal about the value for both of us in sitting in contemplative silence, a healthy and life-giving withdrawal from relating that restores balance and injects oxygen into our existence. Corbett, critiquing the relentlessness of the relational approach, argues that "all of this relating is killing us, as it places an untenable demand on both patient and analyst alike, and risks crowding out the dreamy leisure of reverie" (Corbett, 2014, p. 640). He urges for us to remember, alongside the interaction and self-disclosure, the quieter modes of "being-contemplating-unknowing-reflecting" (Corbett, 2014, p. 638), and the development of "the capacity to be alone" in the presence of another that offers the potential for play (Winnicott, 1958).

There is much to be said for contemplative silence, for containing and waiting, dreaming, getting lost in reverie, listening for links, wondering about theory, allowing ourselves to step out of the relationship for a moment, noticing that we are feeling lost, and reflecting carefully about when to offer a disclosure of our thoughts, feelings or reveries – now, later in the session, next time, in a few months, or not at all. But even when we are contemplating in our own private space in the presence of another, we are still disclosing. It is impossible for us not to self-disclose through our embodied presence. Our intuitive clients will know or learn what makes us laugh, cry, angry, scared, hopeless, inspired, energised, despondent, hurt, frustrated, tender, thoughtful, connected, distant. "Existentially, just by being in relationship we disclose ourselves… in everything we do or say or avoid doing or saying" (van Deurzen & Adams, 2016, p. 77). We can only have empathy for another human being because we can draw on something of our experience or felt sense of our own humanity. I may not have been through the exact experience, but I have known, explored, and brought into awareness feelings and experiences of grief, loss, betrayal, abandonment, enmeshment, intrusion, withdrawal, aggression, envy, despair, hate, judgementalism, love, sexual attraction, repulsion, joy, fear, alienation, oppression. All of these at different times will be articulated non-verbally and covertly when I communicate empathy, even if I choose not to share my exact experience.

The question is often, therefore, not whether we disclose, but how, when, and why we choose to make a disclosure that is explicit rather than implicit or overt. There is also a difference between secrecy and privacy, the former implying a defensiveness or hostility that entails the therapist shutting themselves down and diminishing possibilities; the latter continues to offer possibilities for creative relating. But too much privacy can also be unproductive or even harmful for both in the relationship. Kuchuck (Oates & Kuchuck, 2016) says that therapists will resonate less with clients if they hide or renounce their real reactions, and that privacy and self-negation can lead to isolation and loneliness for the therapist, potentially leading to burnout and acting out.

The unresolvable dilemma of self-disclosure

This chapter has been a struggle. I have written it and re-written it; left it; contemplated, discussed, and read about self-disclosure; experimented with different types and levels of self-disclosure; carried out informal action research with my clients, students, and supervisees; reflected at depth on my practice; and offered my findings to my students and colleagues in reflective inquiry presentations and workshops. What I have discovered is that there really is no one right answer about self-disclosure. The tension in the chapter's writing reflects the unresolvable tension of therapist self-disclosure itself. It is a constant tension between privacy and transparency (or "analytic discretion", (Kuchuck, 2014, p.xxi)). And we can never truly know whether our discretional decision was the right one. We need to maintain as much privacy as we need in order to feel safe and self-contained and to ensure our clients are afforded the privacy that they need without being intruded upon. But we also need to be free to be transparent and to make space in the room for our humanity. And we must be prepared to take measured risks in our work.

What that risk looks like around our chosen level of self-disclosure is a deeply individual decision and one that is constantly changing and under review throughout our careers and in our differing professional roles. Nobody should be judged for making an ethically-minded decision to either disclose or not disclose to their clients something of their lives and humanity, whatever the unforeseen outcome. Humility is crucial in our decision-making process; remembering that behind the mystical curtain of our role, we are simply an ordinary and extraordinary human being meeting with another ordinary and extraordinary human being. Sharing the reality of our ordinariness and extraordinariness can sometimes be exactly what our clients most need. As long as we never lose sight of that mystical curtain of our role.

Chapter 5

Diagnosis, contracting, and treatment planning

An existential perspective

Diagnosis, contracting, and treatment planning in transactional analysis

The treatment triangle

"Observation is the basis of all good clinical work, and takes precedence even over technique" (Berne, 1966, pp. 65–66). This observation of self and other is fundamental to the phenomenological approach to psychotherapy that Berne advocated. He championed mutuality, open communication, and client autonomy in this observational and dialogic process, yet as a doctor and psychiatrist his medicalised terminology of diagnosis, contracting, and treatment planning seems to be at odds with other aspects of his philosophical approach. In this chapter, I am going to outline the classical and more relational approaches to transactional analysis's (TA's) "treatment triangle" (Stewart, 2007), and introduce my ideas about an existential-phenomenological stance to contracting, diagnosis, and treatment planning that may have similarities with Berne's original intentions.

Ian Stewart's "treatment triangle" explains the three-way interaction between diagnosis, treatment direction, and contracting: diagnosis informs treatment direction, which informs the contract for the therapeutic work. How that "treatment" happens depends on the individual client and their presenting issues, as well as the personal style and methodology of the individual therapist. The therapist uses "therapeutic operations" (Berne, 1961), "empathic transactions" (Hargaden & Sills, 2002), or "co-creative empathic transactional relating" (Tudor & Summers, 2014) to effect decontamination, deconfusion, and expansion of the Adult ego state. For Berne (1961), the ultimate aim was script cure and autonomy (the capacity for awareness, spontaneity, and intimacy), whilst for more relational constructivist transactional analysts (Allen & Allen, 1997; Cornell, 1988; English, 1988; Tudor & Summers, 2014), change has been about creating a new script narrative and finding more constructive ways of being in the world through a different experience of relating with their therapist. In the course of treatment and as more information unfurls or

DOI: 10.4324/9781003475217-7

unconscious processes emerge, further diagnoses may be made, which can change the treatment plan and inform a new contract. Alternatively, if the client is satisfied with the changes made, client and therapist may agree to work towards ending (or Berne's rather harsh and clinical sounding "termination").

Treatment planning in TA

This somewhat prescriptive and linear approach to therapeutic treatment was outlined by Berne in a treatment plan: establish a working alliance, effect decontamination (in group therapy), effect deconfusion (in individual therapy), then a process of relearning before termination. If successful, treatment will have led to autonomy and script cure, with three other stages of cure on the way: symptomatic relief, social control, and transference cure (Berne, 1961). Other transactional analysts have added to Berne's treatment plan with additional stages such as redecision, Parent ego state work, and recycling of old script issues (Clarkson, 1992; Tudor & Widdowson, 2001; Woollams & Brown, 1978). It was also rewritten and reframed by Erskine (1973), who suggested instead six different stages of treatment: defensive, anger, hurt, self as a problem, taking responsibility, parents are forgiven.

Others went away from the linear towards a more circular and "backwards-and-forwards" approach to the therapeutic process, with a relational focus on the therapeutic relationship (Minikin, 2008, 2021) or the two-person "encounter" (Cook, 2023). Many in transactional analysis now see the concept of treatment planning as a misnomer, as we do not see our clients as patients who are ill and therefore need "treatment", nor do we see ourselves as doctors who rigidly "plan" what will happen in therapy to find a "cure". Rather we work together with our clients to see what emerges between us in the context of a real relationship. We allow for a more fluid, radical, and relational approach that focuses on dialogue (Buber, 1923/1958) in the real relationship between client and therapist to help the client form and re-form their life's narrative and find new and more productive ways of being in relationship (Minikin, 2021; Cook, 2023).

Diagnosis in TA

Berne's treatment plan was informed by the therapist's diagnosis about what was not working well for the patient in their life. He used therapeutic operations to hear the client's story and the "four pillars" of TA to analyse the client's difficulties: ego states, transactions, games, and script. Further theories developed in different "schools" of TA (classical, redecision, Cathexis, integrative) that provided a broad range of intrapsychic and interpersonal diagnostic tools for the transactional analyst, including the racket (or script) system, drama triangle, life positions, injunctions and drivers, impasse theory, symbiosis, discounting, passive behaviours, personality adaptations, and relational needs. In America in the 1960s, writing on similar themes to R.D. Laing (1960) in the UK, Claude Steiner and Hogie Wyckoff (1975), developed the radical psychiatry movement in TA, which advocated a socio-political perspective to diagnosis and suggested that oppression and alienation needed to be considered as the root cause of people's distress: "People's troubles have their source not within them but in their alienated relationships, in their exploitation, in polluted environments, in war, and in the profit motive" (Steiner et al., 1969/1975, pp. 3–4). Steiner and colleagues went on to say that "All alienation is the result of oppression about which the oppressed has been mystified or deceived" (Steiner et al., 1969/1975, p. 11). This was echoed four decades later in a relational stance to alienation, when Minikin (2018) suggested that through mutuality and contact we could help awaken the client from the mystification of oppression, this awareness leading to necessary disturbance. Relational connection was then the route through disturbance to mutual understanding and plurality with self and others.

Diagnosis (and ultimately transformation) through the therapist's use of self and the therapeutic relationship was the philosophy and methodology of a relational perspective to TA (Cornell & Hargaden, 2019; Fowlie & Sills, 2011; Hargaden & Sills, 2002). Through the transferential relationship (introjective, projective or transformational transferences, or projective identification), the client could unconsciously communicate their non-verbal early relational difficulties, trauma, or fragmented sense of self, which the therapist could hear, understand, and transform by listening to and tentatively acting on their counter-transference (Hargaden & Sills, 2002). At the same time, contemporary constructivist and co-creative perspectives in TA were focusing more on health rather than the pathology of "diagnosis" and what is "wrong" with the client (Summers & Tudor, 2000; Tudor & Summers, 2014). Influenced by the existential perspectives of phenomenology and dialogic encounter (Buber, 1923; Husserl, 1931/2012), they see a mutual dialogue and a focus on the present-centred "between" of the therapeutic relationship as the methodology and method for the client telling their story, discovering their mutual contribution to unproductive relating, and offering new possibilities for relationship.

Contracting in TA

This concept of shared responsibility for and equal participation in the work was always Berne's intention, illustrated in his philosophy of bilateral contracting for change. The terminology may be unfortunate in that it sounds legalistic – and I prefer to use the term "co-creative agreements", particularly with clients – but the concept is essentially about shared responsibility for the work and is intended to ensure open communication, mutuality, and the client's empowerment. Berne (1966) differentiated between the administrative or business contract that is formed at the start of the therapeutic relationship and determines fees, time, location, cancellation policy, and so on, and the professional or treatment contract that determines the treatment direction and nature of the work client and therapist agree to do. This may be agreed in the first session or may take weeks or months to determine, is regularly under review, and may change over time. Berne also astutely encouraged therapists to look out for the "psychological contract" between client and therapist, the unspoken and often unconscious agreement between them: "You will get better to please me", or "You will be the parent I never had". Charlotte Sills (2006) expanded Berne's three contracts to five levels of contract: contract with the world (e.g., ethics); with the organisation and individual (the administrative contract); with the client regarding developmental outcome (the treatment contract); with the client for a session (the sessional contract); and with the client moment-by-moment (a moment-by-moment or "process" contract (Lee, 2006)). Sills also offered the contracting matrix to differentiate between hard and soft contracts, and contracts that involved self-understanding or no self-understanding, later also discussed by Tony White (2022).

Other transactional analysts went on to develop Berne's ideas around contracting. Claude Steiner (1974) outlined four necessities for contracting: mutual consent, valid consideration (we both receive something from the agreement), competency (of both client and therapist), and lawful object (working within the law and ethics). He also discussed an ethical and legal perspective to contracts, and suggested that sometimes the contract might simply be to "find a contract". Fanita English (1975) introduced the three-cornered contract between client, therapist, and an organisation; Maxine Loomis (1982) suggested "care contracts" (for those who were unwilling or unable to make a change contract); and Mothersole (1996) discussed "no-suicide contracts". White (1999) developed "no-psychosis contracts" and later a "contact contract" to aim for genuineness and humanness (White, 2001). In Sill's (2006) book, *Contracts in Counselling and Psychotherapy*, Mothersole suggested "no-harm contracts", Keith Tudor developed three-cornered contracts into multi-handed contracts (to include a supervisor, for example), Peter Jenkins developed an ethical and legal perspective to contracts, and Ian Stewart discussed outcome-focused contracts. Stewart (2007) later went on to outline contracting for safety through "escape hatch closure", and Eusden (2023) discussed ethical risk and contracting in relational therapy. In an existential perspective to contracting, I introduced the idea of an "encounter contract", involving a mutual commitment to dialogue about the immediacy of the therapeutic relationship (Cook, 2023).

Diagnosis, contracting, and treatment planning in existential therapy

Whilst the relational sensibility to TA has introduced more flexibility, fluidity, tentativeness, and an acceptance of uncertainty, many of the more formal TA approaches to contracting, diagnostic categories, and anticipatory treatment planning do not fit comfortably with an existential-phenomenological stance.

Existential contracting

The existential attitude is one where we come together in an encounter without any agenda or anticipation about what will emerge between us, what the outcome will be, or how either one of us will be changed. Jaspers (1925/1960) advocated a stance of "not-knowing"; uncertainty is a pre-requisite for this kind of relating, with the therapist remaining open to new relational experiences. Hard behavioural contracts (Sills, 2006) – which are less committed to exploratory dialogue and more focused on cognitive-behavioural methods that aim for symptomatic relief and social control (Berne, 1961) – are therefore not appropriate for existential therapy. They may, however, be an initial starting point for therapy before transitioning to a more existential stance, and can co-exist alongside any of the other contracts on the contracting matrix.

The contracting matrix

All four treatment contracts on the contracting matrix are helpful to empower the client in thinking and talking through what they want from therapy and the therapist, and whether they wish to work behaviourally, psychodynamically, co-creatively, or existentially – or more usually in a longer-term therapy, a combination of the four. Sills (2006) differentiated between contracts that are hard (behavioural or clarifying) or soft (exploratory or growth and discovery contracts). She also separated them into contracts where there was already self-understanding (behavioural or growth and discovery) and little or no self-understanding (clarifying or exploratory). In this way she accounted for the existential and unconscious psychodynamic struggles of which we are not yet aware, and the uncertain, emergent nature of dialogue and mutual exploration. She also helps us to think about the fluidity of contracting, acknowledging the movement between the various types of contracts with different clients and at different phases of therapy, and in this way such contracting helps therapist and client work together to determine the changing treatment direction, rather than it being planned by the therapist.

From an existential perspective, our professional contract is always held lightly, with the initial contract a starting point rather than an end goal. A hard clarifying existential contract, for example, may be helpful when assisting someone who has enough self-understanding to know that they are suffering from death anxiety. As they learn to tolerate their anxiety, they might transition into a softer growth and discovery existential contract to find ways of making their life more vital and meaningful whilst they are still living. A soft exploratory contract may be the initial contract for someone who does not understand what is making them so unhappy in life, which may lead to working psychodynamically in the transferential relationship to help them integrate a fragmented sense of self. Alternatively, or additionally, they may work co-creatively in the immediacy of the therapeutic relationship with an existential tension around intimacy and withdrawal in relating. With greater self-understanding, they may transition into a soft growth and discovery contract where they want to use the therapeutic relationship more explicitly to develop in their capacity for intimacy. A growth and discovery contract is usually an existential contract. For example, they may be wanting more from their life, perhaps a search for meaning and purpose in a new life stage (such as entering the workforce, moving in with a partner, parenting, the mid-life transition, or retirement).

The encounter contract

An important aspect of existential contracting is what I call an "encounter contract". In our first sessions, I ask new clients what they would like from therapy and from me as their therapist. I also let them know my thoughts on how our relationship and what happens between us can be significant aspects of the therapy. I explain that engaging with the immediacy of our encounter can provide useful information about themselves, their presenting struggles, their worldview, and their ways of relating, and that working through any challenges between us can offer new transformative relational possibilities. In particular, I invite them to let me know if they are experiencing any difficulties or disappointments in our relationship, if I have upset them in any way, or if they are having any feelings about me or the therapy – good or bad – that are challenging or stirring. In doing so, I offer them the possibility of an "encounter contract". This proposes an engagement in dialogue, in the present moment, about our relationship.

Some may need and be striving for this level of intimate encounter from the beginning of therapy, but for many, it may be too threatening or invasive in the early stages. They may need me to enter the lived reality of their disturbance and work psychodynamically in the transferential relationship for many months or even years before they can start to engage with me less as a projection and more as a human being. In these situations, attempting to talk about the immediacy of our relationship can be intrusive and feel more about my agenda than about theirs. However, their capacity for intimate connection will often grow over time as trust, courage, and a more cohesive sense of self develops, and as the work transitions from a focus on psychodynamic disturbance into existential predicaments, tensions, and here-and-now relatedness. Bringing up something about our relationship and tentatively engaging with the immediacy of our relating can be a sign of the glimmerings of a new and enlivening phase of our therapy.

Existential diagnosis: encounter and the phenomenological method

The authentic encounter of the existential-phenomenological method eschews diagnosis, specific technique, and theoretical dogma, preferencing attending to

and being with the client. Our ongoing endeavour is authentic, evolving dialogue: two people being open to each other and to themselves in a live, dynamic,
present relationship, where they genuinely listen to what is being said or hinted
at – even in silence – without preconceptions of where the conversation will
lead or a specific agenda or plan for the direction of the therapy. Therapy may
start with monologue or silence, as this is what the client needs or is all they are
capable of, but successful therapies will end with authentic dialogue (van
Deurzen & Adams, 2016). Rather than searching for connections and patterns
that enable us to pigeon-hole our client into certain diagnostic categories,
therefore, this phenomenological method invites us into a place of "un-know-
ing" (Spinelli, 2005) and an assiduous attentiveness. In discussing the reasons
for her training as a psychotherapist, one of my supervisees described herself
as always having been "nosey". With a slight reframe, we determined that it
was an intense curiosity in people that made her eager to find out more about
them and about humankind in general. An innocent and unpolluted curiosity
is essential to working phenomenologically. We combine an attentive curiosity
with a suspension of our own knowledge, expectations, or predictions, and an
openness to discovering the new and as yet unchartered territory of this individual or of wider humanity. We see things with new eyes and as "novel"
(Spinelli, 2015), looking at what we are hearing and seeing afresh like a child
exploring the world for the first time. Husserl (1931/2012) describes this as
putting aside (or "bracketing") our "natural way of seeing" and being intentional in suspending our known conclusions and judgements ("epoché").
Rather than theorising, problem-solving, explaining, analysing, or attributing
causation (which can be a way of alleviating the therapist's own anxiety), the
existential therapist is committed to exploring the client's worldview: their
unique perspective of the world and their beliefs, values, and relationships. We
are curious, listen to what is *actually* being said, notice, observe, and describe
("what" and "how" rather than always needing to uncover the "why").

TA and the phenomenological method

Of course, the "why" is also important for many people in helping them to
make meaning. TA theory revolutionised my life by helping me to make links
between my past and present, and it was having my eyes opened to the "why"
of my relational dynamics and my own thinking, feeling, and behaviour that
inspired me to train as a psychotherapist. Yet in the early years of my career, I
still tended to use those psychodynamic theories to inadvertently and unhelpfully pathologise myself (and others). My preference now is thus to see the
"why" as a search for affirmative meaning-making, and contemporary TA
therapy as a way to help clients make meaning of their life story or create a new
and healthy narrative for themselves. A person's script ("existential worldview") is therefore not necessarily pathological, as Berne implied, but an ongoing, dynamic life narrative that may be healthy or unhelpful, and an attempt to

come to terms with life's meaning and existential realities (Heiller & Sills, 2010). Berne's version of script as pathology, and his medicalised terminology in diagnosing and treating that pathology, however, was in contradiction to his otherwise fundamental belief in the phenomenological method. He spoke about the therapist having a "Martian frame of mind" (Berne, 1972, p. 444) that enabled distorted perceptions ("Earth-talk") to be eradicated. His suggestion was to have an innocent and embodied way of listening to the familiar becoming strange: "to see the other person as a phenomenon, to happen to him and to be ready for him to happen to you" (Berne, 1972, p. 5). Deaconu's description of Berne's "Martian" is clearly phenomenological: "Looking at the world afresh, harnessing a discourse freed from preconceptions and that remains primarily descriptive as well as vigorously grounded in the realm of the phenomenological" (Deaconu, 2020, p. 194).

The therapist's knowledge, experience, and wisdom

We cannot eradicate diagnosis and treatment direction completely though, nor would I want to. It is not enough simply to describe and clarify, the client needs to understand the meaning of the description for them and make sense of how their experiences are their own personal and context-dependent response to a situation or relationship. By using the content and process of the sessions and the relationship between therapist and client, the therapist can help the client make meaning and form connections to give them a more coherent self and world view. Our knowledge, experience, and gained wisdom enables us to confront effectively, with our own unique way of relating, the client's worldview or script. Every intervention is based on our personhood, our worldview or script – and the history of our life, work and studies – and offers the possibility of new directions by seeing the world and relationships in a different light. Because of our knowledge and experience, we may be able to see in our client's struggle some of the universal tensions with the givens of existence and common existential themes that they are unable to see in themselves. We may also recognise unconscious, disowned "sedimentations" and "dissociations" – or the contaminations and confusions of Parent and Child ego states – that defensively aim to maintain the safety of their worldview or script, and keep them stuck or resistant to challenge. This is at the cost to some aspect of life and self. Van Deurzen and Adams provide a marvellous illustration of sedimentations, that also beautifully describe fixated and archaic aspects of our Child and Parent ego states: the "sediments of the river of life fall to the river floor and give us an increasingly solid but illusory sense of identity that dams up our life" (Van Deurzen and Adams, 2016, p. 68). Whilst not explicitly diagnosing these sedimentations and confusions, we can help our clients make meaning by offering our observations of their predicaments and our experience of our mutual relational struggles, always verifying with them whether this holds true for them.

The dimensions of existence and the holistic self

A form of diagnosis in existential therapy is recognising and identifying different existential themes, tensions, and givens of existence that the client may be grappling with. I explore these below and in later chapters. It is important that we have reflected on these universal issues for ourselves so that we can recognise and tolerate them in our clients and in our relationship. There will always be some existential tensions that we personally struggle with more than others, and having awareness of this through our own depth reflection and relational personal therapy is crucial. It is not about removing the struggle, it is about learning to tolerate and understand it, and finding ways to understand and work productively with the unease in others. For example, I can feel a tension with isolation and exclusion. I know as far as I am able where this comes from in my historical family relationships and my position in the family as youngest child with several significantly older siblings. This generally helps me tolerate the tension between isolation and connection better in the present. There are times, however, particularly in a group, when it is particularly hard for me to feel isolated, and I find myself becoming increasingly dysregulated. This may emerge because of the universal existential tension between group and individual needs or, as is more often the case, when the other I am relating with has their own struggle with responsibility or intimacy. Perhaps having been responsible for others' wellbeing too early in life, or suffocated in a relationship, they may fear taking responsibility for the other and withdraw or refuse to engage. Our interlocking existential tensions around connection and isolation, intimacy and withdrawal, and responsibility and freedom, may then lead us into an unproductive fight-flight or withdraw-chase dynamic. Identifying through honest and authentic dialogue where we are struggling together is a form of co-created diagnosis.

Whilst we always want to uncover existential issues – or any form of "diagnosis" – *with* our clients not *for* them, it is helpful to think about what we might be looking for. I think about this in terms of existential givens, existential themes, the dimensions of existence, and interconnected holistic aspects of existence. All human beings will grapple at different times with one or more of the *givens of existence*: death, isolation, choice, freedom, anxiety, guilt, responsibility, paradox and the search for meaning (Yalom, 1980; Spinelli, 2015). People will also struggle in their own individual way (because of their unique personality and personal history) with any of the *existential themes* around love, hate, safety, belonging, competition, envy, grief, justice, cruelty, kindness, courage, luck, values, punishment, power, or forgiveness. It can also be helpful to consider the *dimension of existence* in which they are having difficulties: personal, physical, social, or spiritual (van Deurzen & Arnold-Baker, 2018). Finally, I suggest thinking about our clients' *interconnected holistic aspects of existence*. Explored more fully in the chapter on the erotic, I see nine different inter-related existential contexts in which we have capacity to connect holistically to self, others, the environment, and the transpersonal: the relational, emotional, intellectual, physical, powerful, sensual, spiritual, sexual, and creative. If any of these are avoided or in tension in life, the person may not be living as fully, erotically, and vitally as they have the potential to do, and this may inform the direction of our work together. Of course, some people do not want to change; it is their prerogative to choose whether they want to live a full and expansive life. In these circumstances, existentially-oriented enquiry and confrontation can help clients identify and take responsibility for these choices, even if we might consider them restrictive.

Existential treatment planning: phases of therapeutic encounter

Any of these aspects of self and relating may emerge in the changing, dynamic, and erotic therapeutic encounter. We need to be attentive to all aspects of a person's holistic being and, rather than aiming for psychodynamic change (or "decontamination" and "deconfusion" in TA) as the ultimate goal and prize of therapy, relate with an openness to what presents itself in the dialogue. Heidegger (as cited in van Deurzen & Adams, 2016, p. 223) differentiates between "leaping-in" (where the therapist takes over the client's autonomy for finding their own direction in life) and "leaping ahead" (where they are respectful of the client's autonomy, helping them wake up to their own potential and revealing new possibilities for their future). That said, there are commonly recognisable phases in a psychodynamic, co-creative, and existential therapy that it can be helpful to acknowledge and reflectively consider (Cook, 2023). Not to *plan* a direction, but to recognise and name what is happening in the work and between us, and to consider if there is anything we might be non-consciously avoiding. The therapist might then offer to their client observations of where they are in the work and what they realise they are not talking about. Whilst not always figural between us, each phase will be implicitly present throughout the therapy and will offer potential for change through the therapeutic encounter. Phases of therapeutic encounter that I have commonly recognised include:

1 Developing the therapeutic alliance
2 Co-creative agreements (contracting)
3 Decontamination and deconfusion (psychodynamic change)
4 Difference, disturbance and impasse (intrapsychic, interpersonal, contextual, and existential)
5 Existential predicaments (death, isolation, choice, freedom, responsibility, anxiety, guilt, paradox, meaning)
6 Erotic encounter
7 Meaning-making (spiritual encounter)
8 Ending

Like planets that revolve around the sun moving closer then further away, these encounters are dynamic and become more or less figural in the therapeutic relationship at different times. There is a beginning and ending of the therapeutic relationship, but otherwise there is no linear pattern; each phase may be visited and revisited time and time again in the client's quest for meaning-making, and some phases may never be explicitly engaged with. In the following case study, I describe and discuss the ebb and flow of different phases of encounter with my client, Martha, and show how an existential perspective to diagnosis, contracting, and treatment planning can be used in a therapy that moves uniquely and almost imperceptibly between psychodynamic, co-creative, and existential relating.

Martha

Developing the therapeutic alliance and initial contracting

Referred to me by her doctor after a medical diagnosis for depression, Martha moved painfully slowly, looked dishevelled, and could not really talk or look me in the eye, let alone make a specific contract for working together. All she could say was that she needed help: she sometimes wanted to die to escape the pain of life, and had a supply of painkillers stored up at home "just in case". She didn't know what help she needed, so I agreed to be with her and to help her in any way that I could, trusting that a route forward and a sense of meaning would emerge for us as our relationship developed. I saw this initially as a contract for support, and we built the alliance predominantly in silence in our early sessions as she seemed gradually to take energy and comfort from my embodied presence. Moment-by-moment contracts were all that she could manage, probably because that was the basis on which she currently coped with life. I occasionally checked in with her: "Is being in silence together helpful?" or "Would you like to tell me anything about what's going on for you?" Usually, she just nodded or shook her head, never raising her gaze from the floor, the wringing of her tightly clasped hands on her lap the only bodily communication of pent-up energy. The poem, "Fear", that evokes the fear of the river about to enter the sea (popularly attributed to the Lebanese poet, Khalil Gibran) came to mind. I wondered curiously what we might discover lurking in the depths of Martha's riverbed. I had no plan, but focused on paying attention to her body's communication and my embodied and emotional responses to her presence.

Disturbance and impasse

From early on, I invited Martha into moment-by-moment and encounter contracts where, with her nodding agreement, I would share with her my observations about our relating, or what her body was communicating: "I notice there seems to be a lot of energy in your hands", or "I'm feeling quite sad as we sit together". I was so used to sitting in silence that I was shocked when, several months into our therapy, she started to talk. "I feel so guilty about my children", she offered suddenly one day, still looking at the ground. "Do you want to tell me about that guilt?" I responded gently. She proceeded to tell me of her regrets about her depressed withdrawal from her young children, and envy and subsequent guilt that that they were more attached to her husband than to her, yet she resented their demands when her depression took all her energy. "So, you feel both guilty and resentful", I summarised non-judgementally, aware of feeling in my body her internal tension of both unexpressed anger towards herself and her children. Martha nodded her head and I noticed her shoulders relax a little. "It looks like your shoulders are letting go of something," I fed back to her. "Yes," she responded, "I think it's a relief to tell you how I feel." The immediacy of the dialogic encounter can help to disrupt or confront the other's worldview, enabling the emergence of conscious and non-conscious stuck places; disturbing feelings and experiences; and intrapsychic, interpersonal, and existential impasses. Starting to face and tolerate these disturbances was bringing Martha a sense of relief. For the first time, she glanced up at me and I smiled as our eyes briefly met. Trying to normalise the existential impasse and paradox of both love and hate, I offered a self-disclosure: "I think guilt and resentment – even hate are very normal feelings when you're a loving mum. I certainly still feel them all – and my children are now in their 20s!" I caught a glimpse of a smile as Martha's gaze returned to the floor, and I noticed that her hands had stilled slightly. We sat in a warm silence for a while. "Would you like to explore your guilt and resentment some more?" I eventually enquired. "I think that would probably be helpful", she agreed.

Exploratory contract and meaning-making

In agreeing to an exploratory contract, Martha and I were going deeper into the uncertainty of dialogue. There was both an anxiety and an excitement starting to emerge in our interactions, a healthy tension in therapy because of not knowing what new aspects of ourselves and life will unfold. Tolerating this existential tension can be helpful in growing our capacity for the uncertainty and paradoxes of life. I stayed genuinely curious about Martha's hidden depths, ready to be surprised by her rather than imposing on her any thoughts around diagnosis. Kaye (1995) describes the process of therapy as a co-creation of novel meanings via mutual dialogue; by being willing to "stand beside" Martha in the telling of her story, we could search together for new meanings and new outlooks on the world.

Over time, Martha described her beliefs from a young age that being a mum would make her life complete, yet with each child she had been disappointed that she still did not feel whole. Gradually she could see that the worldview of her life's "river" had become increasingly polluted by sedimentation: the dam of depression had become a defensive strategy for her to manage the pain and disappointment of the realities of life. She did not feel the extent of the pain, but neither did she experience the vitality of free-flowing life. Through our dialogue, Martha started to realise that her depression was the worldview or script that was giving her a sense of certainty, continuity, and structure, albeit whilst also restricting her. It seemed to feel easier for her to feel guilty about the depression, rather than experience the life force that it quashed. In an attempt to clarify the impasse, I gently challenged her: "So does the depression lead to guilt, or the guilt lead to depression?" I asked. Martha's body recoiled in her chair as my confrontation hit a nerve in a way I was not expecting. After a long period of silence, she almost whispered, "I think it's both".

Decontamination, deconfusion, and de-sedimentation

Our dialogue over the next months oscillated between investigations into her past, present, and future, sometimes within the same session. We spent many months exploring Martha's vicious cycle of guilt, resentment, and depression, and the painful impasses that this left her contending with. She experienced life as disappointing and futile, felt guilty that she was not more satisfied, retreated from her guilt and emptiness into depression, then felt guilty for what she was doing to her children and that she was not making more of her life. Retreating further into herself and her depression to avoid the pain, she cut herself off from a relationship with herself, her children, and her husband, resenting them and herself for the isolation and disconnection, then becoming overcome with guilt and shame for her hateful and destructive feelings. The "soul death" of depression and isolation seemed preferable to her excruciating difficulties with life's connections and lack of meaning.

The confrontation of my presence was integral to our work together. By being an embodied witness of her struggle, I offered the challenge for Martha to come to see and know herself more. She could not completely escape into her isolation because, even without words, I was with her and seeing her, and this was simultaneously terrifying, soothing, and captivating. Having a supportive and gently confronting witness to her distress helped to gradually loosen Martha's impasses and organically decontaminate and deconfuse her split-off or warring ego states. By gradually connecting more with me and with her archaic grief, there was also a de-sedimentation of her dissociative isolating archaic relational experiences. She grieved the alienation she had felt as an only child with parents whose enmeshed and symbiotic relationship had frequently left her feeling desperately alone. Almost simultaneously we explored her current existential feelings of isolation, and the disappointment in her own parenting of her own children. She grieved that her idea of motherhood had proved to be a fantasy, and the hole this had left in her perspective on life's meaning and purpose. She was gradually making meaning and recalibrating her worldview, opening up potential for new possibilities.

Rupture and existential tensions

Despite considerable progress, after some months I began to feel that we were stuck in the sludgy mudbanks of Martha's grief, and I noticed I was moving from empathy to irritation. I wondered whether Martha was being held back by sediments of unexpressed anger, and clumsily disclosed my irritation in an attempt to investigate. Martha withdrew into a simmering silence, clearly hurt and feeling objectified, and in return I felt like I was being punished. This silence lasted for weeks, and I found myself feeling increasingly controlled, hurt, and frustrated, resenting her presence and wanting to end the therapy. I wondered if this was also how Martha was feeling, but she would not engage in exploration. We were touching on each other's sedimented river floors, and the river of our relationship was well and truly dammed up. Feeling disturbed, I sought solace in an exhibition of wildlife photographs from the Natural History Museum in London. I was struck by my magnetic draw to the beautiful, funny, and awe-inspiring, and my physiological repulsion to the pictures that showed animals in pain or taking their last breaths, particularly if their injuries had been inflicted by human beings. I thought about Martha, and how I felt both polarities with her at times, and no doubt she felt with me. Yet both attraction and disturbance were part of the natural world, both part of existence – even the cruelty. I bought two postcards for Martha of photographs that had stood out to me: A funny one entitled *"Forest rodeo"* (A. Ohshima, 2024) of a macaque who had just jumped spreadeagled on to the back of a deer, and the other entitled *"The face of the persecuted"* (N. Aldridge, 2024) of a terrified fox with a mauled face who had been ravaged by hunting dogs. At our next session, I gave her the postcards and told her of my insights. She was clearly touched that I had been thinking about her, and I sensed the erosion of some of our sedimentations. The photographs helped us to begin to talk about the disturbing anger and cruelty that was part of both of us, as well as the kind, beautiful, funny, and companiable. The river of our relationship started to flow again as our rupture enabled us to bring to light our existential struggles with the polarities of seemingly irreconcilable tensions. Finding a creative way to breach the dam and face into life's inevitable conflict with Martha invited a more open and truthful worldview, and greater acceptance of imperfection in life and relationship.

The erotic and an encounter contract

Following our repair, Martha noticeably began to change. Her stance straightened, I noticed a sparkle emerging as our eyes met more frequently, and even an occasional giggle as we shared a joke. Love and excitement were stirring as we experienced the tremors of Martha's erotic life force or "physis" (Berne, 1947). For the existentialist, erotic aliveness is indistinguishable from existence and is about an innate sexuality ("being sexual" (Spinelli, 2015)) or spirituality: a transcendence of time, human relating, life, and death (van Deurzen & Arnold-Baker,

2018). Our sexuality and spirituality are fundamental aspects of our human existence, and a spiritual and erotic connection is therefore ever-present in the therapeutic encounter, even if at times it feels deadened. It is therefore vital to notice and nurture the precious shoots of life when they start emerging. "It feels like something is changing between us, Martha", I observed tenderly. "Yes," she responded coyly. "it's like time is standing still for us and I feel butterflies in my tummy". In this "small second of eternity" (Quinodoz, 2010), Martha was springing into life and responding to my invitation into an encounter contract. I believe our spiritual and erotic connection was enabling her to communicate her aspiration for existence through growth, healing, creativity, recognition, and connectedness. Our encounter was therefore validating Martha's existence and her life force. Expressing our simultaneous anxiety and excitement, shame and desire about our growing intimacy enabled Martha to tolerate better the joys and disappointments of relationship, whilst celebrating her existence in the erotic encounter was a way of helping her choose to live.

Ending: death and life

Where there is life, however, death is never far behind. One day, Martha disappeared. She cancelled two sessions at short notice, then sent an email to thank me for everything, but saying that she wanted a break from therapy. I racked my brains to remember any possible rupture; had I pushed her too hard and she was retreating from intimacy? I invited her back to talk it through – or at least to end well – and told her of my concern that we had experienced a rupture of which I was unaware. She replied that there hadn't been a rupture, she was just enjoying living her life, and wanted to see if she could sustain that without me. She told me again how much our relationship had meant to her, and said, "It's not an ending, I'm sure we will see each other again soon". I never heard from Martha again. For some time, I felt concerned that in not having a good ending we had avoided Martha's death anxiety and the "movement-towards-death" (Heidegger, 1927/2010) that every change, transition or ending symbolises. I was worried that I hadn't been able to help Martha face death without becoming overwhelmed by it, knowing that this is so important to help people live life more fully, authentically and meaningfully (Becker, 1973). I remembered my fleeting thought in our first session about the river trembling with fear before entering the sea. Was she too scared of the ocean of death to face our ending? I was reminded of another photograph from the wildlife exhibition that had haunted me, entitled "The Dead River" (Joan de la Malla, 2024). It was a shocking view of one of the world's most polluted rivers in Jakarta, Indonesia, that is leading to widespread subsidence and the sinking of the city. I thought about Martha being like that dead river when she came to therapy, but realised that she had left with a much clearer free-flowing current. Perhaps she had been so consumed by death that she did not want or need to focus on it through our ending; perhaps it had not been anxiety of death that had deadened her river, but anxiety of life, and she wanted to stay in the river rather than think about the ocean for a while. Possibly, in not saying goodbye to me, she was also keeping me as a life buoy – a way of holding on to life in the same way that her box of pills enabled her to hold on to death. Maybe rather than avoidance, this was in fact Martha's ingenious and creative way of embracing the greatest paradoxical tension of all: keeping both death *and* life as possibilities.

Martha's story and our therapeutic encounter is unique, but I hope it offers some ideas as to the creative use of contracting, diagnosis, and treatment planning in a therapy that combines psychodynamic, co-creative, and existential ways of working together. The therapeutic relationship is like a river that shapes both client and therapist as it flows. The dialogic encounter erodes, transports, and deposits in a way that we cannot diagnose, decide, predict, or plan. We can simply agree to be present for each other on the journey. With mutuality of presence, dialogue, and co-creative agreement – rather than rigid diagnosis, treatment planning, and contracting – we organically wind our way through the different phases of this unique river's course. In doing so, we create distinctive and beautiful landforms, valleys, bends, and lakes – and occasionally ride a waterfall or burst its banks. The only thing we can be sure of on this journey is that the river will eventually become part of the ocean: for all of us, death is a certainty. But with courage, we can take hold of an infinite number of expansive possibilities as the river of life flows its own individual course towards the sea.

Section 2

The development of the adult

Chapter 6

The developmental model of adulthood

The tasks and conflicts of adult life stages

Change and continuity

A process of becoming

My dear 90-year-old mum has dementia, her ways of relating with herself, others, and the world are constantly changing, being de-stabilised, transforming. She is not the same person as she was. And yet there is a continuity about her old self that at times restores some balance and equanimity, particularly when we can still laugh together. Recently, she asked me "is Rachel coming today?". "I am Rachel, Mum", I replied gently. "You can't be", she said, looking incredulous and a bit mischievous, "you're far too old to be Rachel!" In laughing together, I was able to find a connection with the same person that has been my mum for 54 years. Yet she has also changed, to the point where she did not recognise the woman that I had evolved into. I wondered who "Rachel" was for her in that moment. The baby she gave birth to? The five-year-old going to school? The 18-year-old teenager leaving home to go to university, the young woman in her 20s getting married, becoming a teacher, having children? The woman in her 30s becoming a psychotherapist and raising children, or the middle-aged woman in her 40s getting divorced, becoming a single mum, and a teaching and supervising transactional analyst, or in her 50s becoming an author, grieving her children leaving home, and celebrating becoming a great-aunt (seven times over and counting!). Throughout the changes and at all ages I've still been Rachel. I have the same body as the day I was born, yet every day it has changed and continues to evolve spontaneously and imperceptibly. Despite decades of therapy and training, I still have ingrained in me, helpfully or unhelpfully, some of the fundamental, implicit, somatic relational patterns and ways of being-in-the-world and being-with-others (Heidegger, 1927/2010) that I believe have been with me since the womb and will continue to be with me for life. I carry my childhood with me – implicitly, somatically, unconsciously – and yet I am constantly changing, developing, and growing with every relational interaction and life experience: accumulating senses of self, and shedding old senses of self. I am not the same person at 54 as I was as a

DOI: 10.4324/9781003475217-9

school child or bride. I am not the same mother to young adults as I was to them as children or adolescents. I am not the same psychotherapist as the day I graduated, the same teacher and supervisor as when I passed my teaching and supervising transactional analysis (TA) exams. Yet I am still mum, psychotherapist, teacher, supervisor. Life is a paradox of both change and continuity.

I think of the simultaneous change and continuity in Claude Monet's 19 paintings of the Houses of Parliament in London from the early 1900s, painted from the same view but at different times of the day and in different weather conditions. He wrote to his dealer, Durand-Ruel: "I cannot send you a single canvas of London ... It is indispensable to have them all before me, and to tell the truth not one is definitely finished. I develop them all together" (Metropolitan Museum of Art, 2024, "The Houses of Parliament"). The result is a stunning collection of similar but different views, colours, textures, landscapes, and perspectives that is deeply symbolic of our adult development. Like Monet's paintings, we are never completely finished: we carry with us our earlier selves and life experiences, yet we are also an ongoing work of art in the process of development. We are continually – until we take our last breath – integrating past, present, and future. Heidegger (1927/2010) sees this as a continual process of "becoming" throughout life, rather than an end point where we finally "become". Balancing, tolerating, and embracing the ever-present tension between the polarities of change and continuity is a life task to be negotiated for every human. We need to come to terms with the fact that change – wanted or unwanted – is constant and unavoidable: the greatest paradox about change is that it is the only constant in our lives (Spinelli, 2015).

Difficulties with change

It is change that often brings people into therapy or consultation: wanting healthy change, struggling with unwanted change, resisting change, desperately seeking change that is not possible, anxiety about future change, the uncertainty of change. This is often accompanied by defensive reactions that help people cope with change by minimising, avoiding, or denying its impact, but that result in them living less fully and authentically. Spinelli (2015) describes three types of inevitable and continual change. "Spontaneously accepted changes" are unconscious and imperceptible changes that we integrate into our lives every second, hour, day, and year without thought and reflection (our cells dividing or dying, an impactful relational encounter that changes us without our knowing). More noticeable and obviously impactful are "reflectively accepted" or "reflectively troubling" changes. Those changes in our lives that we can reflect on with awareness and that enthuse, disturb, excite, shake, move, and/or surprise us, whether positively or negatively. We can meet reflectively accepted changes head on, albeit with them sometimes having a significant impact on our lives. In contrast, reflectively troubling or rejected changes (or our inability to bring about wanted change) are those that cause the most difficulties in adult life because they are considered unfair, unwanted, intolerable, unacceptable, inflicted upon us: changes such as trauma; loss and grief through bereavement, divorce and relationship breakdown; redundancy and unemployment; infertility and miscarriage; chronic illness, accident or disability. Even positive, desired changes can cause difficulties for there is always a loss involved in change. When things change, we have to give up our old self and ways of being-in-the-world, which can cause anxiety because we do not know who our new self will be. As Robert Kegan suggests, "All growth is costly. It involves the leaving behind of an old way of being in the world. Often it involves, at least for a time, leaving behind the others who have identified with that old way of being" (Kegan, 1982, p. 215).

An existential perspective to change

Sometimes the struggle with these changes is because of psychodynamic disturbance and intrapsychic impasse, but many times the wrestle is an inevitable and unresolvable existential impasse, part of the inherent difficulties of human existence: loss, suffering, death, endings, meaning-making, isolation, anxiety, freedom, and responsibility. Often the struggle is with both. Yet TA has focused almost exclusively on psychodynamic disturbance and the promotion of healthy change. There has been an emphasis on "cure", of redeciding unconscious childhood script "decisions", of providing a reparative experience for people wounded in childhood, or the learning of more productive ways of relating to self, others, and the world through the transferential relationship or the here-and-now therapeutic relationship. This intense focus has come at the cost of considering an existential perspective to the *unchangeable* aspects of human existence, and the *inevitable* changes that occur through the organic lifelong development of the adult throughout every stage of life. My aim in introducing an adult developmental-existential approach into TA is to offer an alternative perspective to the concept of change. To acknowledge that not all therapy is about seeking intrapsychic and interpersonal psychodynamic change, but that it can be about helping people face the inevitability of change, the impossibility of some changes, and the existential givens of a changing life throughout all of the adult life stages. We need to be flexible enough to adapt our stance and ways of working to each unique client and to each of their stages of life and phases of therapy. As Mary Baird Carlsen argues:

> When we respect the vast permutations of adult life, we will be more likely to honor the complexity of individuals and the dialectic between stability and change, between the universal and the unique, and between the internal experience of the person and that of shifting relationship.
>
> (Carlsen, 1988, p. 79)

Change, continuity, and development in TA: ego states

What are ego states?

Eric Berne gifted us with an excellent visual and metaphorical theory for understanding change, the development of the human personality, and each person's intrapsychic and interpersonal ways of being: ego states. They are TA's "foundation stones and its mark. Whatever deals with ego states is TA, and whatever overlooks them is not" (Berne, 1970, p. 243). Thus far, despite Berne's view of TA as an existential philosophy, ego state theory on life development has emphasised psychodynamic stages of childhood development rather than accounting for existential-developmental change and growth throughout adulthood. I later offer a simple ego state model that sees human development in stages from conception to death, rather than simply in childhood. Before I do, I offer a basic introduction to some of the existing ways of thinking about ego state theory.

Our Parent, Adult, and Child ego states are different aspects of our personality and sense of self that have developed helpfully or unhelpfully throughout childhood and that determine (consciously or unconsciously) our thoughts, feelings and behaviour. Berne (1961) described the contents of our ego states as both current and historic, giving a rather dry definition of ego states as "vividly available temporal recordings of past events with the concomitant meaning and feelings which are maintained in potential existence within the personality" (Berne, 1961, p. 19). Whilst sometimes contradictory, Berne generally saw the Adult ego state as about here-and-now, present-centred processing that enables us to draw consciously, constructively, and creatively upon our past experiences. As we grow in awareness, we integrate previously unconscious and historic aspects of our Child and Parent ego states into our here-and-now reality, thereby growing in health and autonomy (our capacity for awareness, spontaneity and intimacy (Berne, 1964)). For Berne, our Parent ego states include unconscious introjects of historic parent-figures and their messages, judgements, and prejudices. Our Child ego states are the unconscious archaic fixations from past experiences, stresses, and traumas. When a person is thinking, feeling, or behaving from their Child or Parent ego states they are, outside of awareness, repeating the past and experiencing themselves "rubberbanding" (Kupfer & Haimowitz, 1971) back to childhood or embodying a past parent-figure that they have unconsciously "borrowed".

Different theoretical views on ego states

Somewhat confusingly at times, Berne described both positive and negative aspects of Parent and Child ego states, such as assertiveness, authority, and nurturing in Parent, and playfulness, spontaneity, and creativity in Child. There is an ongoing tension in TA about whether healthy lifelong development is situated in the Child ego state (Cornell, 2003), all three ego states, or just in the Adult ego state, with unhelpful "pathology" being in Child and Parent ego states (integrated Adult (Erskine, 1988); integrating Adult (Tudor, 2003)). Tudor describes development in a continually expanding, integrating Adult ego state, "which characterises a pulsating personality, processing and integrating feelings, attitudes, thoughts and behaviours appropriate to the here-and-now – at all ages from conception to death" (Tudor, 2003, p. 201). Others (Blackstone, 1993; Clarkson & Fish, 1988; Cornell, 2003; Goulding & Goulding, 1979; Hargaden & Sills, 2002) consider that ongoing growth and development throughout life is shown in dynamic, visceral, affective, and somatic Child ego states that are both regressive *and* progressive vital systems of lifelong mental organisation. Aldridge & Stilman (2024) develop Hine (1997), Allen (2000), and Cornell (2003) in viewing our core self outside any ego state models. Such earliest means of learning and mental organisation exist on sub-symbolic, bodily and affective levels which "developmentally precede the capacities of the ego and underlie/accompany/inform/shape/color the nature of the Child, Adult and Parent ego states throughout the course of life" (Cornell, 2003, p. 34). There is also tension between whether TA methodology and method should be aimed at Adult–Adult, present-centred intersubjectivity (Summers & Tudor, 2000; Tudor & Summers, 2014), or whether we work psychodynamically within the transferential relationship (Fowlie & Sills, 2011; Hargaden & Sills, 2002), using the self of the therapist to hear the unconscious communication of implicit, affective, somatic, subsymbolic processes, and relational experiences of pre-verbal Parent and Child ego states.

Navigating tensions, conflict, and contradictions

The interesting, beautiful, and sometimes challenging thing about these theories is that there are potentially as many views about ego states and how to work as there are transactional analysts! Isn't this evocative of Monet's paintings? We can be looking at the same view but see it in a multitude of perspectives. And just like the existential tensions and contradictions of life, this can simultaneously feel invigorating, growthful, inspiring, and exciting, whilst also feeling frustrating, unnecessary, confusing, and even dysfunctional. These differences of opinion (and sometimes outright conflict!) about ego states and human development emanate from the contradictions inherent in Berne's writing at TA's conception – the protocol level of development of TA and its original system of organisation, learning, and motivation that has endured throughout its lifetime. Like every human, Eric Berne was developing his personality and his ideas throughout his too short career, and he died with contradictions still in place. Won't this be true for all of us?

Navigating our way through conflicting theoretical propositions is much like the negotiation of life's tensions, holding two polarities at the same time and becoming increasingly able to move fluidly between those extremes and through every other point on the continuum. Personally, I do not think it matters which ego state model we use to understand our earliest unconscious processes and our lifelong development. It is possible – and desirable – for us to acknowledge and tolerate the tension of conflict, holding differing perspectives, uncertainty, and the inevitable accompanying existential anxiety. The important thing is that we consider the development of the adult as well as that of the child, whichever ego states (or not) we picture this in. For our development in life is about both integrating fragmented Child ego states, challenging unhelpful Parental introjects, *and* accumulating adult senses of self with every new relational or life experience. Like Monet and his paintings, we are "developing them all together".

Developmental theory in TA

Development in childhood

What has been missing in the colourful diversity of TA's ego state theory has been thinking in greater depth about how the adult develops throughout life. Interpersonal neuroscientific research (Schore, 2019; Siegel, 2020) has provided evidence for lifelong neurological development through relationship – albeit at a slower rate in adulthood than during adolescence – and yet there has been a far greater focus in TA on child rather than adult development (Berne, 1961; Clarkson, 1992; English, 2003; Hargaden & Sills, 2002; Levin-Landheer, 1982; 2003; Mellor, 1980; Schiff et al., 1975). Hargaden and Sills' (2001, 2002) ego state model of the development of the self (pictured in the Child ego state and based on Stern (1985)), for example, describes the accumulation of senses of self and "ways-of-being-with-others... [that] remain with us throughout the life span" (Stern, 1998, p.xi). Hargaden and Sills place Stern's four interrelated senses of self (emergent, core, intersubjective, and verbal) into a developing ego state structure: the emergent sense of self in C_0 (sensory experiences in utero up to two months); the Core self in C_1 (sense of self distinct from other gained from adequate attunement, two to six months); and intersubjective self and verbal self in A_1 (sense of self with other, gained through adequate interaction, connection, and communication, around seven to 15 months). Their focus is on psychodynamic disturbance of these senses of self in early childhood and the deconfusion of the Child ego state through the therapist's use of their own self, whilst working in the introjective, projective, and transformational transferences (based on Kohut's (1971) self object transferences of mirroring, idealising, and twinship, and Moiso's (1985) projective and introjective transferences). Whilst this is a helpful psychodynamic theory, what they do not address is the continued growth and accumulation of senses of self throughout adulthood. They also do not offer a methodology for working with the existential dilemmas of adulthood, where growth can be about coming to terms with the existential givens of life rather than simply resolving psychodynamic disturbance.

Development in adolescence

Some TA authors (Barrow, 2014; English, 2003; Levin, 2015; Levin-Landheer, 1982; Newton, 2006) have moved beyond childhood development to argue for the significance of development in adolescence. They suggest that adolescence is a major period of transition, meaning-making, and development of the self, when childhood issues are recycled at new levels of sophistication. Fanita English's (1977, 2003) cumulative model of childhood development, represented like the cross-section of a tree trunk in successive concentric circles in a Child ego state, acknowledges the progressive levels and stages of development throughout both childhood and adolescence. Yet she draws an "outer bark" to represent the integrated Adult surrounding the child and adolescent ego states, suggesting that growth and integration of personality is complete after adolescence. Pam Levin (2015) also saw the task of adolescence as forming a unifying "skin" around the three ego stages formed in childhood, enabling the integration of the ego states into a cohesive, whole adult personality, whilst Novellino (2008, p. 235) argues that we can achieve a "fully functioning Adult ego state" through resolution of unconscious conflict in (male) adolescence.

Development in adulthood

These views discount the full potential for lifelong development of the self. I personally balk at the idea of aiming for a cohesive, whole adult personality, or a constrictive "bark" of adulthood. It feels suffocating, stagnating, and stifling. I do not want to be restricted to being the same person at 90 that I was when I was 18, 25, or 50, or whatever age someone suggests that adulthood should be completed by. Even Berne, in his typically contradictory fashion, advocated for a "biological fluidity" (Moiso, in Erskine et al., 1988, pp. 9, 12), a continual development throughout life shown in healthy growth of all three ego states over time. Whilst there will inevitably be physical and cognitive decline for us all, we surely have lifelong potential for psychological, emotional, and spiritual growth until death. In TA, this is perhaps best shown in Pam Levin-Landheer's (1982; Levin, 2003) "Cycle of development", which suggests that we revisit stages and "powers" of childhood (being, doing, thinking, identity, being skillful, regeneration, recycling) in more sophisticated ways in adulthood:

> Like the stages of growth in all nature, the patterns of adult life are cyclic, seasonal and based on a continuation of the stages of growth in childhood. We return to certain themes and issues over the course of time. We grow through the physical and emotional changes typical of each stage in childhood, then go back again and again.
>
> (Levin-Landheer, 1982, p. 129)

This recycling in adulthood (in contrast to a linear and progressive approach to meaning-making) is echoed by Cornell (2003). He suggests that the organising, motivating, and learning principles of Child ego states are rooted in the earliest stages of life and endure and circuit back throughout the lifetime, living and changing in the present and informing, shaping, and helping us make meaning from birth to death: "Rarely in psychotherapy do we create new patterns of emotional and relational processes for the future without first circuiting back, if even briefly, into memories of the past..." (Cornell, 2003, p. 37). The constructivist-developmental psychologist, Mary Baird Carlsen (1988), offers a similar view in her meaning-making perspective to adult development. She suggests that our lifelong developmental task is about the working, reworking and deepening of our meaning-making – or our script narrative in TA terms: "The adult story develops through solution and resolution of old problems seen in the light of the new" (Carlsen, 1988, p. 77). For me, this implies both a recycling of the old, with a movement into something new: development is both cyclic *and* linear or progressive. We carry our protocol and childhood experiences with us somatically, intrapsychically, and interpersonally; it is part of the narrative of our life, our identity, and our being-in-the-world. But we also accumulate *new* senses of self across the lifespan from conception to death, we do not simply rework old ones. We always have the potential to expand and develop as we progress anew throughout adulthood. As T.S. Eliot (1943) suggested in his poem, "Little Gidding", we are continually exploring but the end of our exploration will be arriving where we started and it being as if we see the place for the first time.

Integration of different approaches to change

Perhaps in TA the concept of the adult's continual growth is best represented by Co-creative TA (Summers and Tudor, 2000; Tudor and Summers, 2014). The philosophy of Co-creative TA is based on ongoing growth through present-day relating rather than on exploring lifelong regressive or progressive unconscious processes. However, it only touches lightly on the unconscious, and is unfortunately limited in linking past, present, and future and offering an existential perspective to the struggles, tasks, developmental stages, and conflicts of adulthood. I think we need an integration of all these different approaches, philosophies, and methodologies: progressive and regressive unconscious processes; psychodynamic disturbance; present-centred authentic relating; and an existential-developmental perspective to adult growth that accounts for the universal hopes, concerns, struggles, tensions, choices, responsibilities, and anxieties that every adult will encounter as they transition through different life stages. We need the courage, reflexivity, and flexibility to work in different ways with different clients and at different times, and to hold in a multitude of ways the potential for change – and the acceptance of things that we cannot change. We need to be open to the possibility that not every difficulty in life emanates from psychodynamic disturbance in childhood, and see change in terms of helping our clients make their own meaning of their life, form the ongoing and evolving narrative of their lives, and to help them navigate the conflicts, challenges, meanings, and tasks of adult life that shift and fluctuate as we transition through different life stages.

A new ego state model of adult development

To help us conceptualise this adult development, I offer a simple ego state model to illustrate the progressive accumulation of senses of self throughout the lifespan that is not currently represented in other ego state models. I adapt English's (1977) concentric circles from her childhood model of development to include ongoing evolution into adulthood. Rather than a fixed outer bark after adolescence, I view death as the fixed end point – when growth (in this life at least) is complete. Until then, and throughout adulthood, there is a pulsating and expanding outer edge to represent ongoing psychological, spiritual, and existential philosophical growth throughout life: "A developmental perspective honors the fact that even though a person's body is wearing out, human awareness, understanding, and wisdom can continue to evolve until the end of life" (Carlsen, 1988, p. 76).

With my focus on adulthood, I picture development in an integrating Adult (Tudor, 2003) ego state rather than English's model in Child, but you can equally represent this lifelong development in a dynamic Child ego state that expands throughout adulthood if this makes more sense to you. Ideally, there would be an infinite number of possible concentric circles, as every relational and life experience continues to change us psychologically and spiritually. But, like life itself, we are faced with the limitations of finitude in attempting to diagram the complexities of the human being! I therefore draw on adult developmental psychology research to simplify our lifetime growth into eight different life stages: infancy, childhood, adolescence, emerging adulthood, early adulthood, middle adulthood, mature adulthood, and late adulthood (see Figure 6.1). Each stage builds on our foundational core somatic and organismic self (Cox, 2001) and the enduring relational themes of our childhood that are ever-present throughout each life stage.

Core self

To live authentically, we need to understand how our life development is true to, or in conflict with, our core self. This has been described variously as the "real self" (Berne, 1972), the "true self" (Clarkson, 1992), or the "organismic self" (Rogers, 1953). Aldridge (2021) described it as the seat of bodily urges and hungers, instincts and physis, continually present over time, that encompasses our unique core identity, characteristics, qualities, and "nature" endowed since birth (including our race, sexuality, and neurodiversity): "the

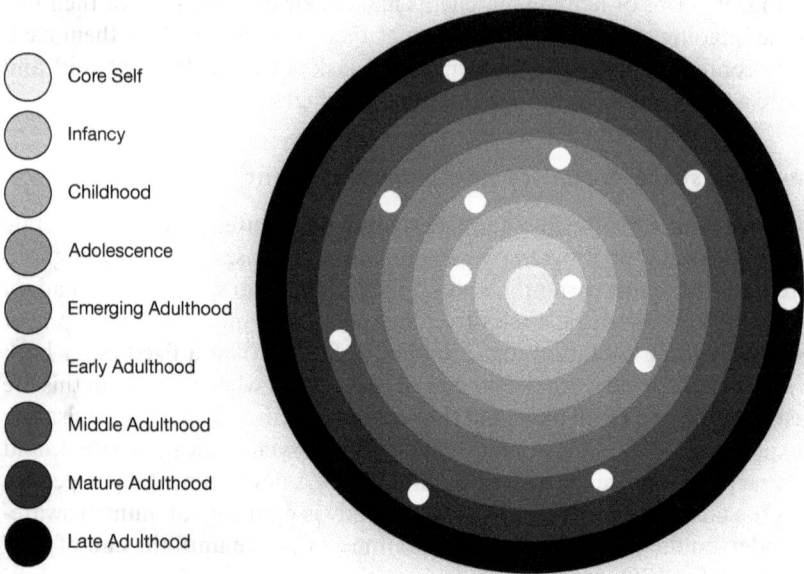

Figure 6.1 The eight life stages and the core self.

paper or slate on which our experience is written" (Aldridge & Stilman, 2024, p. 52). I think of this as our "soul", the erotic, spiritual, and sexual core of a person, the inner being where desire and potential for growth and creativity resides. It is part of us from conception to death (and possibly into eternity), whether or not we live authentically and congruently to it. Buber describes this as the "Oneness of Desire" that precedes the "I–Thou" connection: the "powerful, world-begetting Eros" that is "mediator of the pollination of being" (Buber, 1965, p. 28). This is the foundational spiritual life force of every human being on which our lifelong developing "sense of self" (Clarkson, 1992), "feeling of self", or "moving self" (Berne, 1972) is founded throughout different life stages.

When our developing sense of self and core self are congruent, we can be said to be living authentically in our "whole self" (Berne, 1964). We receive adequate support through the difficulties, traumas, and misattunements of every life stage and can make meaning of them and integrate them into our authentic sense of self. I illustrate this with the "knots" in each life stage; just as in a tree, where living wood grain grows around wounds in the trunk, our vulnerabilities form unique curves that make us more distinctive and beautiful. Experiences of unsupported alienation and trauma (and the accompanying emotions or affect) can be introjected, split off, and sequestered away in Parent and Child ego states throughout life, resulting in new decisions and meanings that result in our living inauthentically and at odds with our core self. Our work through every life stage is to help people make meaning of their past and current experiences in such a way that their sense of self (or "moving self") can become more authentic to their real or core self.

Aldridge and Stilman (2024) see the core self as situated outside the traditional ego state model: ego states develop as we form a sense of self. I prefer to see our core self at the centre of our being and at the heart of the Adult ego state, present from the conception of our existence and throughout life and an illustration of our "existence preceding essence" (Sartre, 1943/1956). Our "essence" develops as we constantly imagine and reimagine our identity, natures, and values over time: "Man first of all exists, encounters himself, surges up in the world – and defines himself afterwards" (Sartre, 1946/2007, p. 28). In other words, the human being we become – our identity – is chosen by us as we make meaning, through development in different life stages, of our embodied existence in our historical and cultural context. It is these stages of life, and the conflicts, challenges and tasks of different life stages, that I suggest we consider when being alongside people in their process of making meaning and "becoming". Before delving deeper into each life stage, I offer a brief summary of the adult developmental psychologists and existential philosophers and psychotherapists whose work has inspired me.

A brief history of adult developmental psychology

Sigmund Freud and Carl Jung

Developmental life stages were first considered in psychoanalysis by the Austrian founder of psychoanalysis, Sigmund Freud (1905), who described development in terms of childhood psychosexual stages. He believed that personality was developed in the first five years of life, with psychological problems in adulthood resulting from the lack of resolution of conflicts and traumas in these childhood stages (oral, anal, phallic, latent, and genital). He believed that we can become stuck or fixated in certain stages, leading to unconscious conflict around sexual desires and aggressive impulses. Carl Jung (1931/1970), the Swiss psychoanalyst, psychiatrist, and psychologist, disagreed with Freud's focus on sexuality as a key motivating behavioural force, and described instead the influence of a psychic energy or life force, of which sexuality could be one potential behavioural manifestation. Unlike Freud, he also saw life developing throughout adulthood. He used the metaphor of the sun sweeping across the horizon to think about life in four stages: Childhood, Youth, Middle life, and Old age. "In the morning it rises from the nocturnal sea of unconsciousness and looks upon the wide, bright world which lies before it in an expanse that steadily widens the higher it climbs in the firmament" (Jung, 1931/1970, p. 397).

Erik Erikson

Freud's psychosexual stages of development and Jung's life stages were developed by the German-born psychoanalyst and psychologist, Erik Erikson (1950, 1968). Having moved to the US in the 1930s, he worked with Eric Berne and was a significant influence with his thinking on script, ego states, autonomy, games, and psychobiological hungers. Moving away from psychosexual development, Erikson (with his American wife, Joan (1997)) outlined eight life-long stages of psychosocial development with their own individual challenges and conflicts, the negotiation of which help form our identity: infancy (trust vs mistrust), early childhood (autonomy vs shame/doubt), play age (initiative vs guilt), school age (industry vs inferiority), adolescence (identity vs confusion), young adulthood (intimacy vs isolation), adulthood (generativity vs stagnation), old age (integrity vs despair). Unlike Freud, who described our inner conflicts as unconscious and our identity determined in the early years of childhood, Erikson considered many of these conflicts to be conscious and resulting from a lifelong developmental process. He suggested that a satisfying life depended on successfully negotiating these conflicts in each of the life stages, and, in doing so, developing associated personality strengths and qualities such as hope, will, purpose, competence, fidelity, love, care, and wisdom (Erikson & Erikson, 1997). The end goal, for Erikson, was ultimately achieving integrity and wisdom in old age.

However, when Joan Erikson (Erikson & Erikson, 1997) reached her 90s after Erik's death, she realised the naivety of their views about old age and said that the resolution of conflict in this later stage of life was not about reaching unattainable integrity and wisdom but about spiritual development and coming to terms with the dystonic polarity of each of the previous life tensions: mistrust, shame, guilt, inferiority, role confusion, isolation, stagnation, and despair. Similar to Tornstam's (2005) "gerotranscendence" (a psychospiritual developmental theory of positive ageing that offers a transcendent perspective on time, space, life, and death), Joan Erikson said that successful ageing in this late stage of life was about humility, a greater focus on what is above and beyond, and a redefinition of the self in relationship to others and the universe.

Robert Havighurst

Writing about the stages and tasks of life at the same time as Erikson was the American scientist turned experimental educationalist and expert on human development and ageing, Robert Havighurst (1972). He proposed that human development can be thought of as a process of moving through stages from infancy to older adulthood, with each stage having age-specific developmental tasks around relationships, career, economic standard of living, family life, caring, leisure, values and ethical systems, integration into social groups, civic and social responsibility, and adjusting to ageing. He proposed that it is the successful attainment of these tasks that leads to approval by society and happiness and success in achieving subsequent tasks. He described "teachable moments" in life (Havighurst, 1972), where an individual's life situation means they have a greater readiness to learn and apply information.

Daniel Levinson

Also influenced by Erik Erikson was the American adult developmental psychologist, Daniel Levinson (1978, 1996). He conducted in-depth interviews to form his life stage theory of dynamic "seasons", differentiating between men and women and highlighting the alternating periods of stability, crisis, and transition throughout life: pre-adulthood stage; early adulthood transition; early adulthood stage; midlife transition; middle adulthood stage; late adulthood transition; late adulthood stage. He emphasised the particular challenge of the transition periods (when two eras overlap), and, like Havighurst, went beyond psychosocial development to explore the various developmental tasks of adulthood (around home, career, family, community, ageing) that need to be mastered to progress from one era to the next.

George Vaillant

Two additional stages to Erikson's model were added by George Vaillant (2002, 2008), a leader in the field of positive developmental psychology in America. Through longitudinal studies of adult development, he included "Career consolidation" after Erikson's young adulthood (intimacy vs isolation stage), and "Keeper of the Meaning" after Erikson's middle adulthood (generativity vs stagnation stage). He highlighted the correlation between successful ageing and educational level and physical health, and, like Havighurst and Levinson, he conceptualised stages of adult development more as tasks of adulthood: developing identity and intimacy, career consolidation, generativity, becoming keeper of the meaning, achieving integrity. He claimed that his model was descriptive of successful ageing rather than predictive, and encouraged a focus on the essential positive human skills of affection, compassion, forgiveness, and wellbeing, rather than simply on anxiety, depression, and stress. This was developed by the positive psychologist, Martin Seligman (2011), who saw human development as building positive character strengths such as optimism, creativity, self-regulation, self-determination, integrity, and wisdom.

Bernice Neugarten

Perhaps the pre-eminent authority on ageing in the twentieth century – and particularly accounting for cultural differences – was the pioneering adult developmental psychologist, Bernice Neugarten (1968, 1979). She was the first to conduct research on personality and ageing, and became hugely influential in helping to change public policy in the United States against ageism and towards "intergenerational equity". She found that personality develops slowly with age and over the lifetime, rather than being fixed in childhood, and additionally highlighted the wide diversity and fluidity in ageing between both individuals and cultures. Her "social clock theory" (Neugarten, 1968, 1979) highlighted the implicit and explicit cultural expectations of age-appropriate behaviour, and that adult personality change was often determined by the adherence to or divergence from their culture's social clock (Berk, 2023). Neugarten argued for a fluid life cycle, not one determined by a chronological age, with psychological themes and preoccupations of different life stages appearing and reappearing in different forms throughout life rather than fixed in a single life stage. This is reminiscent of Pam Levin-Landheer's (1982) "Cycle of development" in TA, which suggests that we recycle certain powers throughout life: being, doing, thinking, developing identity, being skillful, regeneration, and recycling. Importantly, Neugarten argued that age was a bad predictor of a person's health and ability to function. She challenged many of the stereotypes of middle age (the mid-life crisis, menopause as necessarily traumatic, and empty-nest syndrome), and differentiated between the more active, independent "Young–old" (which I call "Mature adult") and the less able, dependent "Old–old" (which I name "Late adult").

Robert Kegan and Lisa Lahey

Also moving away from seeing life as a progression through stages or about the gathering of new information or skills was the trailblazing American constructivist-developmental psychologist, Robert Kegan. He expanded into adulthood Jean Piaget's (1971) cognitive developmental stages of childhood, seeing development as an ongoing process of lifelong evolution and transformation: "A person is not a stage of development but the process of development itself" (Kegan, 1982, p. 219). He described the self as a "restless creativity" (Kegan, 1982, p. 1) that is "an ever-progressive motion engaged in giving itself a new form" (Kegan, 1982, pp. 7–8). For Kegan, life *is* motion, rather than merely something *in* motion, and our adult development about an evolution of consciousness and increasingly complex ways of knowing. Transformation is therefore about changing the form of our mind by making meaning and updating the way we perceive and understand the world. Kegan believed that transformation is necessary to transition to higher stages of development, but that this comes at a cost and needs courage because crisis and tragedy are often the catalyst for such growth. Kegan & Lahey (2009) outline five levels of cognitive, emotional and subject-object relational stages of development and evolution: the "impulsive mind", the "imperial mind", the "socialised mind", the "self-authoring mind", and the "self-transforming mind". Each stage builds upon the previous one and few adults progress through all stages in their lifetime.

Like Levinson's transitions, Kegan and Lahey describe the vulnerability of the evolutionary "balance" of moving through each stage, and that "to understand another person in some fundamental way you must know where the person is in his or her evolution" (Kegan, 1982, p. 114). Life's evolution starts with Stage 1 in childhood, the "impulsive mind": primarily egocentric, concerned with their own needs and desires, with limited capacity for empathy and controlling impulses. Stage 2 (adolescence and emerging/early adulthood) is the "imperial mind": a more ethnocentric stage, where the individual identifies strongly with their social group, family, tribe or nation and often conforms to group norms. Stage 3 (which Kegan and Lahey speculate is reached by about 58% of the adult population and I link to early/middle adulthood) is the "socialised mind". This is a more world-centric stage of development, with a greater capacity for empathy and openness to diversity, and the ability to question societal norms. Stage 4 (speculatively reached by approximately 35% of the adult population and which I picture in middle/mature adulthood) is the "self-authoring mind". This is a more inner-centric stage where the individual develops a strong sense of self, adaptability, and personal values, and is able to hold their own beliefs whilst respecting others' viewpoints. Finally, Kegan and Lehay say that only about 1% of the adult population develop to Stage 5, the "self-transforming mind" (which I picture as mature/late adulthood). This is more integral or global-centric, where individuals have more of a holistic worldview and seek interconnectedness and commitment to personal and societal growth. They understand that multiple ideologies can coexist, are more comfortable with ambiguity and paradox, and are able to hold contradictions, polarities and multiple perspectives. I see this as a more spiritual perspective, perhaps likened to Rogers' (1963) "self-actualization", whereby one is closer to reaching their potential and able to believe in the unique potentialities of others.

Mary Baird Carlsen

This more existential-developmental perspective to ageing was also presented by the American writer and developmental-constructivist psychologist, Mary Baird Carlsen (1988, 1991). Like Kegan and Lahey and existentialists such as Viktor Frankl (1946/1969), she brought a meaning-making perspective to the lifelong, ongoing, and dynamic process of creative ageing. She focused less on biological chronology and more on the potential for lifelong personal growth through the search for meaning. Carlsen (1988) said that examining contradictions in life through conversation and debate in a developmental dialectical therapy could help the individual reach a higher truth, enabling the emergence of the individual from the "dark wood" to a "place on the mountain":

the movements from crisis to resolution; from endings to new beginnings; from the unnamed to the named; from limbo to finding one's way; from the experience of being within the problem to standing outside the problem with new perspectives and understandings… the movement from meaninglessness to meaning.

(Carlsen, 1988, p. 4)

For Carlsen, developmental transformation in adulthood emerges through interactive relationships, whereby old difficulties can be recycled into something new. She was influenced by developmental psychiatrists and psychoanalysts, Calvin Colarusso and Robert Nemiroff, who suggested that the person's movement into new contexts and relationships throughout life help to restructure their perspectives on self and others: "The fundamental developmental issues of childhood continue as central aspects of adult life but in altered form" (Colarusso & Nemiroff, 1981, p. 67).

Carlsen suggested that we cycle through Erikson's eight stages of psychosocial development in miniature – from trust to intimacy to generativity to integrity – with every new context or relationship. Nothing is every resolved once and for all, and the developmental processes in adulthood are influenced by the adult past as well as the childhood past because every situation and trauma leaves an imprint upon the human personality (Colarusso & Nemiroff, 1981). Like Kegan, she saw dangerous opportunities of crisis being the opportunity for constructive change, and rather than an emphasis on diagnosis, treatment, and symptom reduction, she therefore aimed to harness the energy and emerging health of the crisis experience. Like van Deurzen & Arnold-Baker's (2018) fourfold encounters of existence (the physical, social, psychological, and spiritual), Carlsen (1988) had an appreciation for the spiritual developments which can occur with age and the overlapping systems within the human being – the physical, social, emotional, cultural, communal, cognitive.

The stages, conflicts, and tasks of adulthood

In the next chapters, I draw on these authors' work and my own personal and professional experiences to bring a new adult life stage theory into TA. I stipulate from the beginning that the ageing process is individual, fluid, and culture-specific, with everyone developing in different ways and at different speeds. It is, of course, impossible to describe a person's uniqueness or their distinctive evolution into any life stage theory, and I do not wish to define anyone by their life stage. The limitations of developmental theory are described well by Kegan:

> The stages, even at their best, are only indicators of development. To orient around the indicators of development is to risk losing the *person developing*, a risk at no time more unacceptable than when we are accompanying persons in transition, persons who may themselves feel they are losing the person developing.
>
> (Kegan 1982, p. 277)

Whilst acknowledging that there is no blueprint of life (van Deurzen, 2012), I think it can be helpful to consider common patterns of the stages, conflicts, challenges, and tasks of adult life as we accompany our clients in finding their own meaning and wisdom. In each of the subsequent chapters on individual life stages, I address, through case studies and lived experience, some of the common tasks and struggles I have observed and encountered that are particular to that stage. Sometimes this struggle is with the complex and disturbing existential tensions and inevitable givens of human existence: life and death; aloneness and relatedness; love and hate; freedom and responsibility; choice, change, and time; existential anxiety and guilt; spirituality, and a search for meaning. I do not suggest that any existential struggle is solely or even primarily the concern of one particular life stage; we all negotiate these human tensions in different and developing ways throughout life. I have simply seen these struggles emerge or significantly shift for myself and for the clients about whom I write.

I do not set any agenda for the chronological ages of each stage, nor do I want to impose my meaning on them or try to make people advance through the life stages in a way that I may think appropriate. Some people will navigate every stage in their lifetime, others will never reach late adulthood because of death, denial, or being unable to maintain the mental and physical youthfulness of middle or mature adulthood. Others will reach late adulthood but will miss out development from other stages. We can visit, re-visit, and skip stages, and return to tackle some of the tasks of the earlier stages at a later time of life.

Cultural differences

We must remember the significance of culture for people's outlook on the stages, conflicts, and tasks of life. What I may consider a "task" of a certain stage of life may be completely different in another culture. Social class, religion, ethnicity, and cultural heritage will determine opportunities, values, and beliefs about the nature of life and its different stages (such as marriage, raising children, caring for elders, gender roles, work, and further education). My perspective cannot help but be that of a privileged British, White, heterosexual, cis-female, able-bodied, middle-class psychotherapist. I have been raised and live and work in an individualistic society, with its focus on independence and individuation and valuing personal over group development. My country is not currently in the throes of war, my nation is not being oppressed. The challenges of adult life and a search for meaning can be very different for those who are less privileged, who continue to suffer from greater levels of oppression and alienation than I have ever experienced, or whose search for meaning is at an existence level because of very real threats to survival. Even without such threats, those from collectivist cultures often have a different value and belief system from individualists, such as interdependence, social harmony, respectfulness, and group needs over individual needs. With a greater sense of belonging, social support, and connection to the transpersonal, these cultures often seem to have greater life satisfaction. However, they are also associated with lower self-esteem and feelings of mastery (Yetim, 2003). It is vital that we are curious with our clients about how their culture is influential in how they consider the tasks and stages of life, and that we do not impose on them our own personal and cultural value system. Our concern should be for them to find their own way to be authentic to their core self, and to help them find their own balance of autonomy and connection – with their self, others, the environment, their culture, and the transpersonal (Cook, 2022).

Universality

Cultural difference notwithstanding, we all share a basic humanity. There is a universality in the inevitability of existential givens that face us all from conception to death. Considering life stages, tasks, conflicts, and transitions can provide a simple map to help us locate where a client might be struggling or lacking authenticity, which life stages may have been interrupted, and which existential issues they may be grappling with. As the first three life stages – infancy, childhood and adolescence – have been written about extensively in TA, my focus in the next chapters will be on the five broad adult life stages: emerging adulthood, early adulthood, middle adulthood, mature adulthood, and late adulthood, ending – quite appropriately – with chapters on life and death. As I write, I identify with being in middle adulthood. I therefore write with humility about later life stages as I have not yet experienced them for myself. I hope I do. And yet just because I have experienced the earlier life stages does not make me an expert on any of them, for it has been my own personal and unique life journey. I have learnt from observing, being alongside, having others accompany me, reading, soaking up others' experiences. I want to acknowledge and appreciate the many people who have inspired, guided, and accompanied me as we have climbed together from the dark wood to the side of the mountain and back again many times, each time ascending a little further towards the mountain peak with each navigation out of the dark wood. The relational presence and life experiences of my family, friends, supervisors, therapists, mentors, colleagues, students, supervisees, and clients has shown the potential, time and again and in every life stage, for recycling old difficulties into something new, and finding growth from the novel experiences that life thrusts upon us. Each new crisis provides us with new opportunities for personal transformation and evolution as we climb the mountain of life, for as the eminent mountaineer, Sir Edmund Hillary, suggests: it's not the mountain we conquer, but ourselves.

Chapter 7

Emerging adulthood
Entering the adult world

Venturing from home

"Philosophy is really homesickness – the desire to be everywhere at home." This paraphrase from the writing of the twenty-year-old German novelist and philosopher, Novalis (2007), in the 18th century, describes beautifully the cry for home of many young people transitioning into the adult world: the simultaneous cry for security, certainty, comfort, identity, love, freedom, a lost past of childhood, safe challenge, and the life force of venturing into an exciting, unknown future. Whilst a yearning for home is at the heart of the human condition at every life stage (van Deurzen, 2012), those entering emerging adulthood often experience it more intensely. Often not yet feeling a solid internal anchor of identity and integrated life experience, they can be less able than those in later life stages to tolerate an existential homesickness, leaving them feeling lost, alone, and adrift as they peer into the vast expanse of possibilities.

On the day I left school at the age of 18, simultaneously exhilarated and terrified, I remember crying with my mum saying that I didn't feel old enough; leaving school and becoming an adult was something that my older siblings did, not me! Yet it can also be a time of paradox, when the young person feels simultaneously ready and unprepared. Four years after leaving school, at the tender age of 22, I felt so mature and geared up for adulthood that I was indignant that my parents thought that I was too young to get married. Three decades later with the luxury of hindsight, and with my sons now at a similar age, I have a lot more empathy with my parents' standpoint! I was ill-equipped for the adult responsibilities I undertook, and in those exciting and terrifying early years of marriage, mortgages, and career, I often longed for the safety and security of the "home" of childhood.

This tension between feeling ready and not ready, wanting the challenge of venture whilst simultaneously needing the safety and security of "home" is a struggle for many young people transitioning from adolescence into adulthood. Recently leaving to go travelling in Asia, my 24-year-old son, dwarfed by a symbolically enormous rucksack, gave me a particularly tight hug and said

DOI: 10.4324/9781003475217-10

gratefully, "It's reassuring and grounding to be at home before going away". I was struck by his desire for both safety and risk, dependence and independence, home and venturing. Unlike me at the same age, he is discovering his adult identity by postponing full traditional adult responsibilities and instead encountering the freedom and excitement of a world of different possibilities.

The cultural evolution of emerging adulthood

My son's life stage has been coined "emerging adulthood" by the American psychologist, Jeffrey Arnett (2024), a relatively new phenomenon of adulthood. Whilst I and others my generation had often jumped with both feet straight from adolescence into early adulthood (Levinson's (1986) "Early Adult Transition"), Arnett and other developmental psychologists (Sheehy, 2006; Buhl & Lanz, 2007) discovered in industrialised societies an evolving transitional life stage of "provisional adulthood", between adolescence and mid-to-late 20s. In emerging adulthood, full economic independence and adult commitments and responsibilities such as marriage/life partnership, the development of a career, and parenthood are put on hold to enable the pursuit of further education, apprenticeships, travel, creative pursuits, and experimentation in relationships. Whilst acknowledging cultural and socio-economic variations, Arnett (2024) describes five general features of emerging adulthood in industrialised societies: feeling in between (neither adolescent nor adult); identity exploration (especially in love, work, and worldview); self-focused (lacking responsibilities and obligations to others rather than being self-centred); instability (frequent changes in living arrangements, relationships, education, and work); and possibilities (choosing between a multitude of life directions). For those with family or community support that enables the postponement of full economic independence, it is a stage of self-focus, on "being" and "doing" (Levin-Landheer, 1982), particularly in Western cultures where individualism and autonomy is celebrated more than the collective group, family, or community. However, with less privileged socio-economic conditions this life stage is often not accessible because of increased possibilities for dropping out of school, unemployment, little access to vocational training, low-paying jobs, and early parenthood. In developing nations in particular, it is only the privileged minority who experience emerging adulthood, often for a shorter time than their Western counterparts (Arnett, 2024). The overwhelming majority of young people in rural, farm-based, economically-impoverished regions of Africa, Asia, and south America have limited education, and typically enter lifelong work, marriage, and parenthood early. They therefore typically go straight from adolescence (or even childhood) into early adulthood.

Cultural differences notwithstanding, emerging adulthood has developed as a life stage in Western societies because of rising costs of living that make independence increasingly difficult, as well as changing demographics and worldviews, and a shift in the cultural "social clock" (Neugarten, 1979): society's expectations of the timeline of life's milestones. As people live longer, they are having a greater number of long-term relationships and multiple careers (Scott & Gratton, 2021), and societal views on marriage, parenthood, religious beliefs, and career paths are becoming more diverse and less rigid and structured. With the exponential growth in information available through the internet and social media, today's emerging adults are being exposed to a greater variety of novel experiences and a multitude of viewpoints and ways of living. Attitudes towards gender, sexuality, sexual and relationship choices, neurodivergence, spirituality, and work roles are becoming increasingly liberal (Berk, 2023) and today's emerging adults are increasingly able to "individualise" their identities and feel free to change them over time. College, university, training, or a new workplace can be a formative "developmental testing ground" (Berk, 2023, p. 460) for new ideas, beliefs, values, experiences, and worldviews. More than that, when once adult status was recognised by qualifications, career, marriage, and family, research suggests that emerging adults are increasingly seeing the construction of a worldview and a set of beliefs and values to live by as the marker of adulthood (Arnett, 2024).

Challenges of emerging adulthood

When well-supported in their ventures, emerging adulthood can be a time of deep exploration, play, creativity, and growth. New opportunities, the solidification of beliefs and values, and the discovery of an identity that feels authentic to their core self can lead to a sense of flourishing in life, greater self-understanding, and increased self-esteem (Labouvie-Vief, 2006). However, it can also feel like a stage that is neither here nor there: at the age of 21 my younger son described his stage of life as "feeling like life hasn't really started, I'm in a waiting period for something". Worse, it can be a time of angst, guilt, tension, recklessness, depression, and anxiety. Risky behaviour is often a consequence in this life stage: in the US, research has shown that alcohol and drug use peaks among 19–25-year-olds (Berk, 2023), and that a trend towards more sexual partners, "hookups" (emotionally uninvolved, casual sex), and "friends with benefits" (casual sex in an existing friendship) in this life stage often leads to lower self-esteem, regret, risk of sexual dysfunction, and depressed mood, especially for women (Lewis et al., 2012). Continuing to rely on parents can make some feel disempowered, and a fair few can still feel pressured by family, society, or themselves to become independent when they do not yet feel ready. They can feel an existential guilt and anxiety that they are not building their relationships, careers, or families, yet be reluctant to lose their freedom to intimacy and commitment because they are enjoying the newfound feeling of personal control over their lives – perhaps stronger than they may ever experience again. Erikson's (1968) tensions of "Identity versus confusion" and "Intimacy versus isolation" can feel particularly troublesome for the emerging adult.

Existential anxiety

With the continual bombardment of immediate and depressing worldwide news through social media and its selective algorithms, existential anxiety and "Angst" (Kierkegaard, 1844/1980; Heidegger, 1927/2010) – a nothingness, nausea, and anguish – can be painfully and ever-present for the emerging adult. They can fear for their own survival and that of the world because of climate change, nuclear warfare, conspiracy theories, artificial intelligence (AI), global pandemics, and economic crises. They often display a strong sense of responsibility to the world which can bring a positive sense of meaning to their life if they are able to develop proactively a "spatio-temporal outlook" (Spinelli, 2015) and look to a future beyond their own existence without becoming overwhelmed. For some, however, this overwhelming responsibility can cause a paralysing existential fear, and they seek therapy desperate to ease their life-destroying anxiety.

Whilst we can help emerging adults with some cognitive-behavioural strategies for anxiety management, it is important not to view anxiety as something pathological and something to be "got rid of". Anxiety is inevitable when we move from comfort, certainty, and habit into the new, challenging, and unfamiliar, a regular journey for the emerging adult. Our sympathetic nervous system is activated and anxiety arises in the gap between certainty and possibility (van Deurzen, 2010). On one side of the coin is fear, insecurity, and paralysis; on the other, enlivening excitement. Anxiety can thus be viewed as a sign of life and engagement with the world and its infinite possibilities, and therefore something to be normalised and accepted as universal to humankind. We cannot have the vitality of excitement without some anxiety. Schneider (2023) argues that these polarities emanate from birth, when the infant experiences both a sense of groundlessness and terror of the uncontained unknown, alongside a sense of wonder, intrigue, fascination, and curiosity. The tension of the emerging sense of self of the infant (Hargaden & Sills, 2002) is paralleled for the emerging adult. Whether the infant and the emerging adult meet new experiences with anxiety or excitement, or a healthy integration of both, depends on how they are met – historically and in the present – in the terror of their groundlessness as well as the erotic life force of their wonder.

Choice

Like the infant facing multiple new possibilities in life, emerging adults need considerable support with the overwhelming freedom of choice for important life decisions. Without historical or current support, the navigation of choice can make emerging adulthood a particularly stressful time of life. Loneliness, confusion, uncertainty, lack of direction, recklessness, depression, and anxiety can result from the lack of containment experienced with freedom.

Kierkegaard describes this existential paradox as the "dizziness of freedom" (Kierkegaard, 1844/1980, p. 61), whilst Sartre says we are "condemned to be free" (Sartre, 1943/1956, p. 34): existential anxiety is the price we pay for freedom, for consciousness, for deliberation, for engagement with the world, to be able to think about things and find ourselves. For some emerging adults, there is a recklessness in their choice-making and an abdication of responsibility as they resist the transition into adulthood; for others, the overwhelming sense of responsibility and uncertainty inherent in making choices can feel paralysing. They may not have the previous life experience to know that mistakes and regrets are survivable or to understand fully that no one choice will singularly impact the outcome of our lives. It is only through living that we discover that "Life is the sum of all our choices" (Pythagoras, cited in Spinelli, 2015, p. 40): the narrative of our life story is written chapter by chapter throughout our life stages, not finalised in the choices of emerging adulthood. It is not uncommon to see clients in their 30s and 40s still struggling with the choices and responsibilities of emerging adulthood, sometimes presenting as a midlife existential life crisis. These clients have usually not had enough support from parent figures as they enter adulthood. In individualist societies it is often young men in particular who have been left to their own devices, being expected to be independent before they are ready, hide their vulnerabilities from a young age, and programmed not to seek support. Whatever their gender, these young adults can feel alone at sea, adrift without an anchor, compass, or oars, and are still flailing around, decades later, trying to find their bearings and a glimpse of the safety of the shore on which they can land and finally feel grounded.

At whatever age people face head-on their life choices, there is always the potential for loss associated with choice. When we choose, we give up the possibility of the alternatives – what "might have been" – and with loss comes grief to a greater or lesser extent. The possibility of this loss can cause paralysis for the emerging adult who is usually relatively new to significant responsibility for choice. Alternatively, because of childhood trauma they may have had responsibility for choice early in childhood and adolescence, moving into adulthood before their time, and may now rebel against time-appropriate adult responsibilities or need to grieve the impositions on them and the choices they did not have in childhood. Many people come to therapy struggling with situations for which there is no choice, and emerging adulthood may be the first time they experience significant restrictions or have the ability to seek professional support. Life experiences such as disability, chronic illness, relationship abandonment, redundancy, abuse, oppression, work, and educational opportunities are often inflicted upon us because of our facticity – our genetic make-up, intersectional identity, socio-cultural heritage, the situation of our birth, and the family we are born into – or because of others' choices. Even a strong moral or ethical worldview about topics such as abortion, sexuality, or the lifelong nature of marriage can feel like there is no other option because to choose otherwise would involve a fundamental loss of identity. Rather than considering having no choice, Heidegger (1927/2010) prefers to think of it as a "single-option choice", because in these situations, our choice is to decide *how we want to respond* to that which is inflicted upon us. Many existential philosophers and psychotherapists agree: Spinelli says "Choice is not about choosing the stimuli themselves. Rather, our choices lie in how we *respond* to these stimuli" (Spinelli, 2015, p. 40). Rollo May (1969), influencing Berne's theories on transactions, suggests that between every stimulus and response we have a choice, whilst Frankl (1946/1969) says that the greatest mark of a person is how they choose to respond to suffering and make meaning out of it. Jaspers (1925/1960) argues that it is difficulty with coming to terms with life's "limit situations" that causes difficulties for people with single-option choices. Perhaps one of the greatest character developments through the life stages is to come to terms with the unfairness and frustrations of life's limits.

False and passive choices

Often facing life's limit situations for the first time, emerging adults can make "false choices", engaging with fantastical thinking and/or discounting their facticity in the choices they make. One of my disabled clients was persistently applying for jobs that she was physically not able to fulfil, leading to frustration, pain, and resentment on rejection. Our conversations and my empathic confrontations helped her begin to acknowledge and grieve her limitations and take responsibility for making true choices that were authentic to her core self. Passive choices, where responsibility is passed to someone or something else, can also enable avoidance of the pain and anxiety of choice. Emerging adults, as for adults at any life stage, may abdicate responsibility to other people, fate, luck, determinism, fatalism, the Universe, God, their therapist, seeking advice from those who will steer them in their desired course. "I'm going to leave it to fate", "God will do the right thing for me", "the Universe always makes it right in the end", "I can't leave my marriage because of the children". In doing so, we can pass the blame for the outcome on to others rather than risk being responsible ourselves. Our challenge to people making passive choices is that not choosing is still a *choice*; as Sartre (1946/2007) said, there is only one choice that we do not have and that is not to choose. Those who live a fulfilling, proactive, and personally responsible life are seemingly those who have learnt to face up to the limits of existence, their responsibility for the choices they have in life, and who have developed the capacity to tolerate the inevitable anxiety of uncertainty. In taking responsibility for their decisions, mistakes, and losses, emerging adults can learn to make increasingly difficult choices, live with excitement as well as fear, make meaning out of suffering, and with every new experience, learn about what choices they may want to make differently in the future. With such personal development comes a greater creativity in the freedom of imaginative possibilities for the future (Mullen, 1995).

The benefits of therapy for the emerging adult

With emerging adulthood being such a minefield of struggles and possibilities, it is positive that this generation is increasingly open to seeking therapy as a buffering effect against the stresses of this life stage, as well as for personal development and identity-exploration. This generation have suffered from the isolation and social pressures of growing up as "digital natives" (Prensky, 2001), flooded by pseudo-lives and technology-based relationships on social media and video platforming. However, the rise of digital information, artificial intelligence (AI), social media, streaming services, and video-sharing websites has also led to a growing de-stigmatisation of mental health issues for emerging adults and a flood of accessible information and psycho-education. If they can access affordable psychological services (which are sadly still in short supply), I am finding that many arrive in therapy well-informed about relational dynamics and self-help strategies, and are regularly psychologically, holistically, and philosophically-minded with a good understanding of the importance of self-care and expressing feelings. What is often missing, however, is an understanding of how they do this in practice. Gathering information from artificial intelligence and digital "relating", they sometimes have neglected the significance of finding their meaning and identity through the embodied experience of human relationship. Berk argues that "Helping young adults establish and maintain satisfying, caring social ties is as important a health intervention as any" (Berk, 2023, p. 456), and the challenging companionship of embodied therapy can help develop an emerging adult's capacity for relationship. Our provision of the "motherly breath" of home whilst they venture can help them discover home in themselves, others, nature, the world, and the transpersonal.

But a compassionate "home" is not simply soothing, it offers an optimal disturbance and enlivenment that encourages growth. The sacred space of the home of therapeutic relationship allows them to breathe, see the world with a sense of both fear and wonder, and tentatively explore the enormity of the existential givens of life. It offers soothing for debilitating anxiety, encourages an acceptance of inevitable anxiety, challenges the avoidance and pain of responsibility, and celebrates the erotic life force of passionate engagement with the world. Being a therapist for emerging adults (as it is for all struggling adults) is to be a challenging companion; a supportive witness of their explorations; a protector from the terrifying emerging awareness of existential aloneness; a sherpa and guide helping keep them upright and grounded on their challenging climb; and a celebrant of their initiation, curiosity, experimentation, and intuitiveness. In short, our embodied presence welcomes and affirms a young adult's emerging being-in-the-world.

Emily

Emily, a 19-year-old young woman, came to see me in her first year of university. She was lonely, scared, highly anxious, and said that at times she would prefer to be dead than face the depth of her pain. She was desperately homesick, longing for the past security of friends and school, and yearning for a sense of home that she had never really experienced in her childhood. She had found an identity through the structure, academic success, and friendship groups at school, and she felt their loss acutely with the "culture shock" of university and feeling like a very small fish in a very big ocean. She said evocatively that her experimentation with independence felt like she was "dressing up as an adult" and "like being on a rollercoaster without anyone in the control room"; the world felt scary and unwelcoming and she felt like she was teetering on the edge of an abyss, untethered and exposed. Emily desperately clung to others to help her feel protected, lurching from symbiotic relationship to symbiotic relationship in a recycling of old childhood patterns of trauma, yet each time she was experienced as too demanding and clingy and she was rejected, leaving her devastated, anxiety-ridden, and fearing for her survival. Her life-destroying anxiety demonstrated a profound ontological insecurity (Laing, 1960), an insecurity at the core of her being which emanated from a fragile core sense of self, as well as an inevitable existential anxiety of the transition into adulthood. The combination of past, present, and future anxiety was so overwhelming that she was unable to access the erotic excitement of her life force and she was immobilised by the terror of transition into adulthood.

Providing a sense of home

Both her ontological insecurity and her existential anxiety were initially soothed by my stable, often wordless, embodied presence that offered her support, protection, and space. Sometimes she came and sat in silence or sobbed quietly for the whole hour, and I felt like a steadying life raft that she could cling to amidst the storm of her past and present life. The brief respite each week allowed Emily to breathe, my potency offering her a shock-absorber for the stresses of life, and a temporary protection from disappearing into the enormity of her existential aloneness. As Steiner powerfully described: "Potency is expressed in permission ... and is exemplified in protection by the willingness of the therapist temporarily to carry the burden of the patient's panic when in an existential vacuum..." (Steiner, 1968, p. 63). Emily often spoke of the comforting smell of my therapy room, as if she was inhaling the life-breath of a supportive other. It reminded me of the writer and poet, Sylvia Plath's (1967) description, in her poem "The Bell Jar", of the comfort of returning home at the age of 19, the same age as Emily. She described alighting from the train on to the station platform and being enveloped by the motherly breath of her home community as she inhaled the smell of lawn sprinklers, station wagons, tennis rackets, dogs, and babies. Through the sacred, empathically challenging, and potent space of the therapeutic relationship, I was offering Emily that "motherly breath".

Emily later described our silent sessions as being the most profound, helping her to feel more solid, less fragile, and giving her greater courage and inner strength to find a sense of home in herself and to face head-on the existential givens of life. My presence communicated implicitly and silently that I had been through it before, and demonstrated that the terror, despair, and existential angst was survivable. This enabled her to gradually absorb my potency so that she could become solid enough in herself to bear to hold her own existential anxiety. As she did so, our relationship became more challenging and potent, a necessary prerequisite for an effective home. I experienced Emily starting to push me more, challenging me whilst also asking me for extra sessions. I met her challenge head-on, realising her need to tussle to find her potency. I became more confrontational about her passive and false choices, life's limit situations, and the inevitability of anxiety and suffering, and turned down her request for more of me. She was angry and disappointed, accusing me of being uncaring and lacking in empathy. I talked about my slight feeling of suffocation, and challenged her that my "no" was also deeply empathic; what she was facing was an inevitable "limit situation" of life: others would not always be soothing and endlessly available to her, there were limits in even the most compassionate of relationships, and sometimes we have to face difficulties on our own. Our relationship moved to becoming sparring partners; I was a challenging yet supportive companion that she could wrestle with to enable her to start seeing different perspectives and possibilities. Over time, Emily became increasingly able to accept my boundaries and limitations – whilst holding on to my genuine care – which helped her accept more those of life and other relationships (Frankl's (1946/1969) "paradoxical intention"). In doing so, she became far more adept at balancing the tensions of relatedness and aloneness, anxiety and excitement, fear and curiosity, which enabled the opening up of possibilities in her world; she reported thriving in her university studies, social life, and relationships, and tolerated far better the ups and downs of a blossoming romantic relationship.

As Emily approached her graduation and the ending of her university life, her anxiety increased again. She became overwhelmed with the responsibility for the empty expanse of adult life ahead of her and the vast number of choices she was encountering. What career should she choose? Where should she live, and with whom? Did she want to stay in her long-term relationship? Rather than try and alleviate the anxiety, I accompanied her through it and offered her playful challenges about her responses. I suggested that her anxiety was a normal response to this life situation, and encouraged her to view it as a healthy engagement with life and the excitement of future possibilities. We explored together what was important to her to make meaning of life, confronting the contaminations of other people's and society's definitions of meaning. I also helped her grieve for the ending of this period of her life, as well as for the loss of all the possibilities that were no longer available because of past and present choices, and the choices of others. This releasing of energy brought Emily to life; as she tolerated and expressed her grief, anxiety, and excitement, she became more expansive, passionate, and creative about her ideas for her future, and forgiving of her own limitations, those of others, and of life itself. Rather than clinging to me, she was now in charge of her own life raft, better navigating the paradoxical tension of being created by the circumstances of the past and present, whilst being responsible for creating new circumstances in the face of this.

The creativity of emerging adulthood

Emily's unique story of emerging adulthood highlights our inevitable interconnectedness with the world, at few times in life more significant than in the experimental and creative years of emerging adulthood when we navigate the tension of identity versus confusion and intimacy versus isolation. We are all both products of the world and producers of a new world (De Beauvoir, 1948); as Merleau-Ponty writes: "We choose our world and the world chooses us... freedom is always a meeting of inner and outer" (Merleau-Ponty, 1945/1962, p. 454). The emerging adult is facing the meeting of inner and outer as they negotiate the impact of their past; the anxieties, excitement, choices, and changes of their present; as well as the abundant possibilities of their future. This meeting of inner and outer in emerging adulthood was brought home to me recently when visiting the Van Gogh Museum in Amsterdam. Vincent van Gogh's emerging adulthood was spent experimenting – as art dealer, bookseller, schoolmaster, and lay preacher. It was not until he was 27 years old, with the advice and financial support of his younger brother, Theo, that he started painting. Theo's unwavering love and support sustained Vincent through those years of emerging adulthood; when Vincent was 19, they started a lifelong written correspondence which recorded the torment of Vincent's life as he searched for meaning and purpose in adulthood. There is no doubt that it is because of Theo offering Vincent support, protection, and space that Vincent was able to live for ten years with his devastating mental health struggles and fulfil his life's vocation as he transitioned into early adulthood.

At the museum in Amsterdam, the memorial to van Gogh's life's work, I stood weeping in front of "Almond Blossom", the painting Vincent van Gogh had created in a French asylum to celebrate the birth of his nephew, Theo's only son. The beauty, richness, vitality, and depth of the colour, as well as the poignant story around it, touched my soul at a level that is almost impossible to put into words. He did not choose his mental illness and the struggles that he had inflicted upon him, but I couldn't help wondering whether the excruciating agonies of Van Gogh's life enabled that soul-to-soul connection that has been, for so many who have cried in front of his paintings, so wonderfully transformational. Reading some of their letters, I believe that this was possible because Theo provided Vincent with a sense of home – both physically and metaphorically – that sustained him. Providing a sense of home, with its support, protection, space, and challenge, is what we as therapists can do for those struggling to find their life's meaning and purpose in emerging adulthood. In the words of Vincent writing to Theo in 1883, "To save a life is a great and beautiful thing, but it is also very difficult and requires great care. To make a home for the homeless, yes, it must be a good thing, whatever the world may say, it *cannot* be wrong" (van Gogh, 1883).

Chapter 8

Early adulthood

Sculpting the landscape of life

The landscape of early adulthood

Identity and commitments

The emerging adult is like the trapeze artist that has let go of the bars of adolescence and is hanging in the danger, uncertainty and aliveness of mid-air (Tournier, 1972). As they commit to catch the bars on the other side, they swing into early adulthood. This occurs at different ages and in different ways for every person and culture. By the age of 24, I had a husband, my own home, a stable career as a teacher, and an adopted cat; by the age of 30, my family had grown by two children and two cats! Yet despite the security of my external circumstances and identity, it was not until I started developing a stronger sense of self and a greater toleration of aloneness through having therapy in my 30s that I felt that I was reaching adulthood. Sometimes it is the dawning of a new decade that signifies a change in life stage. For C.S. Lewis (2000), the British writer, scholar, and theologian, it was turning 30 when he describes in his personal letters to a close friend the strangeness of realising that he was now coming to terms with being a walking and talking adult. For others it is getting married, becoming settled in a career or becoming parents. The author, Stephen King, in his novel, "Christine", questioned: "Has it ever occurred to you that parents are nothing but overgrown kids until their children drag them into adulthood? Usually kicking and screaming?" (King, 1983, p. 250).

This "walking and talking adulthood", embraced willingly and excitedly or with kicking and screaming, has been described by Levinson (1986) as the settling down period of life, traditionally marked in Western cultures by finding and keeping a well-paid job, forging warm, stable relationships with friends and intimate partners, running a home and finances, perhaps becoming parents, being family and community-minded, and feeling generally satisfied with life. It can be seen as a period of life when there is a merging of Erikson's (1986) tensions between identity and confusion, intimacy and isolation, and generativity and stagnation. Because of the multiple possibilities and commitments of this period of life, it is seen by developmental psychologists as a time of

DOI: 10.4324/9781003475217-11

changing internal organisation and deeper and broader exploration of identity as existing commitments are evaluated. Berk (2023) suggests that the markers of adulthood involve a greater certainty of commitment and the development of knowledge, skills, and various cognitive, emotional, and social attributes: having the ability to plan, using time effectively, making decisions, and reaching goals; building self-esteem, coping strategies, persistence, greater emotional self-regulation, and conflict resolution skills; as well as developing a strong moral character, with a greater sense of personal responsibility, a desire to contribute meaningfully to one's community, and a deeper sense of spirituality, purpose, and meaning in life. Quite a tall order!

Priorities

Many of these markers of adulthood are echoed by existential philosophers, artists, and creative thinkers. Kierkegaard saw adulthood as about finding what it is that you are prepared to live or die for, deciding on priorities, and accepting the regret and anxiety that you cannot do it all. After much soul-searching, Kierkegaard decided not to marry and broke off his engagement in his early adulthood to devote himself to his writing and Christian faith, poignantly voicing the tension of his life decisions: "If you marry, you will regret it; if you do not marry, you will also regret it" (Kierkegaard, 1843/1987, p. 243). The 20th-century English avant-garde sculptor, Barbara Hepworth, who was known for her philosophical linking of art, landscape, and life, chose to preference her artistic work over both relationship and the overwhelm of full-time mothering of four children. Married twice in early adulthood, and with a second open marriage that offered little support, she received significant misogynistic criticism for going against 20th-century British social norms and putting her baby triplets into nursery. She described the tension of her decision to focus on her work, particularly being a woman in the masculine world of sculpture, as feeling like a wounded gull being pecked to death by the healthy ones (Bowness, 2017). Yet sculpture was her identity and remained what she was prepared to live or die for, ironically and poignantly dying in a fire at her art studio.

Change and fluidity

Since then, the 21st century has seen greater openness to freedom of choice for early adults in Western society, as the "norms" of adulthood become less conventional and more fluid. It is now more commonly acceptable to forgo monogamous marriage for life partnership, successive relationships, singleness, or polyamory. There is greater acceptance of fluidity in sexual and gender identity, and people are able to choose to have children in a heterosexual or queer relationship or on their own through adoption and fostering, or surrogacy, sperm, or egg donation. With an increased life expectancy, early adults are increasingly no longer expecting to have a lifelong career but various and changing professions throughout working life (Scott & Gratton, 2021). They are also often acutely aware of how Artificial Intelligence (AI) will impact the nature of employment in their lifetimes, with suggestions that, in time, 40% of jobs around the world will be affected by AI, raising to 60% in advanced economies (Cazzaniga et al., 2024). With a greater focus on gender equality around shared parenting and household responsibilities, and a rise in home-working since the Covid-19 pandemic, many early adults are choosing different working patterns that enable both in the partnership to spend more time with family, hobbies or leisure (Berk, 2023). Greater economic pressures, however, mean that some are unable to afford to buy or rent their own home and are choosing or forced to live more simply or creatively: living with extended family or in less expensive forms of accommodation such as caravans, houseboats, or communities.

Challenges of early adulthood

Loss and disillusionment

Of course, as we have seen, greater freedom of choice is a double-edged sword. Life in early adulthood with a myriad of growing responsibilities, sacrifices, and possibilities can be exhilarating, exciting, and satisfying, but also deeply challenging, stressful, and at times turbulent and anxiety-provoking. On top of the challenges and sacrifices of juggling career, finances, home, parenting, and relationships, early adults can be facing bereavement, redundancy, unemployment, financial difficulties, dissatisfaction with relationships and working life, mental or physical illness or disability, or wider caring responsibilities for parents, grandparents, or other extended family members. Some become disillusioned with life and are grieving the loss of a more care-free, less responsible existence, questioning their earlier life decisions and longing for freedom. "I love my children, but I don't love being a parent", or "I love him but I'm not in love with him anymore" have been laments I have heard on numerous occasions in the therapy room.

Coming to terms with the twists and turns of unexpected and unwanted life events can be particularly challenging. Early adults are often less well-equipped than older adults at coping with the effects of stress and more often report depressive symptoms than middle-aged people, many of whom have attained vocational success and financial security and are enjoying more free time as parenting responsibilities decline (Berk, 2023). Difficulty with making enduring commitments, feeling that the wrong commitment has been made, or a nagging question of "is this it?" can cause considerable distress, leading to anxiety, depression, higher alcohol and drug use, and risky behaviour (Kunnen et al., 2008). Yet deepening financial and relational commitments can make finding an alternative, more satisfying route, seem impossible.

Insufficient support

Early adults need consistent, warm, and appropriate support that also fosters their autonomy, but in an individualistic society, many lack extended family support because of being emotionally or geographically distanced. They may also have less time for social connection outside their partner or nuclear family because of the demands of blossoming careers and family, or simply working long hours to make ends meet. Those in more collectivist cultures might find more support from respected elders, religious leaders, and multi-generational community living, but some might be resistant to seeking support from their social network because of cultural expectations of interpersonal harmony and reciprocal support, or fear of being a burden. Psychotherapy can help the early adult navigate the existential dilemmas and pressures of this life stage, whilst offering a supportive function: a helpmate who has navigated similar routes and can guide them in their exploration of unknown territory, and a cheerleader as they seek widening external support from extended family, friends, work, hobbies, and community networks.

Relationship pressures

Movement into early adulthood often involves a struggle with the shift from "me" to "us", and the shattering of the fairytale fantasies of adulthood. One couple described relationship therapy as having their "bubble burst" as realisation gradually dawned that there is no perfect mythical mate or utopian solution to life's challenges, and that the sacrifices and negotiation of marriage and parenthood are inevitable. Disagreements can often emerge over whether to marry, live together, or have children, or there can be painful dilemmas about whether to end their relationship. Relationship difficulties, affairs, or breakdown can result from the desire for personal change and a quest for new identity; an insecurity, threat, or envy if a partner is developing in a different way to them; or if they feel that their freedom is being restricted. Young adults can also have difficulty adjusting to finding themselves single and/or childless, particularly if close friends and family are moving in different life directions. Even if they are content with their decision to remain single or childless, there can be family and social pressure to conform, and they can feel excluded, misunderstood, or alienated as they increasingly find it hard to find their "tribe".

Parenting

Parenting is, for many, undoubtedly a joy and a privilege, but it has also been the most challenging task of my life so far! In early adult life, those who become parents need – but often don't have – a great deal of support. Parenting is fraught with potential obstacles and predicaments at every stage. The internal and external pressure to have children can feel overwhelming, particularly for women with declining fertility as they age. They may face the difficult and often lonely decision of whether to remain childless or to parent alone. Single parenting – through choice or because of death, divorce, relationship break-down, or accidental pregnancy – is an exceedingly demanding, relentless, and often isolating task, and there remain significant conscious and unconscious biases about single parents that add to the loneliness, particularly for women. Unwanted pregnancy may create intrapsychic and interpersonal tension because of the woman's own ambivalent feelings or pressures from their part-ner, family, religion, or culture, and there may be significant grief whichever decision is made. Infertility can have a significant impact on self-worth, self-es-teem, relationships, and a sense of meaning in life, whilst fertility treatment can be a relentless, intrusive, lonely, all-encompassing, and often devastating roller-coaster. Women can face intrusion to their bodies, relationships, and career opportunities, and partners can feel impotent, pushed out, and objectified. Facing difficult decisions about anonymous donor insemination, surrogacy, or adoption can feel paralysing and terrifying, particularly for single-parents, whilst adopting a traumatised child can create difficulties with bonding and an often explosive, shocking, and discombobulating introduction to parenting, sometimes with regrets and associated guilt.

For those fortunate enough to conceive a wanted child, pregnancy can seem precarious and scary, and it can be challenging to come to terms with their transitioning responsibilities, altering body, and the changes in their partner. Pre- and post-natal depression for both parents is not uncommon, particularly if the road to parenthood has been fraught with difficulties. Sleep-deprivation and exhaustion, little time for self and their partner, physiological and hormo-nal changes, birth trauma for both parents and child, changing levels of attrac-tion and sexual desires, and relational competition, control, and unaddressed resentments can have a damaging effect on sexual and emotional intimacy. Old interlocking script patterns can emerge as they feel rejected, abandoned, suffo-cated, or engulfed, and as they face paradoxical and competing desires around intimacy and withdrawal. There can be conflict about how to raise children, and competition about how to share the parenting and demands of running a home, which can result in a lack of mutual empathy and support. The contin-uing unconscious patriarchy can be destructive to relationships as some women in heterosexual relationships report feeling they carry the mental burden of home and childcare, even if both partners work full-time. A female client described becoming like "housemates" with her partner rather than lovers. Men can feel that it is an impossible and overwhelming burden to be simulta-neously successful in their careers and sharing responsibility for the home and childcare, whilst still feeling a cultural pressure to be the traditional provider and protector.

There is often an extra layer of stress for step-parents in blended families, for those attempting to co-parent with a hostile ex-partner, or when facing parental alienation or fighting for parental access through the legal system. In addition, cultural differences, continuing discrimination, and alienation of parents in the LGBTQ+ community, parenting neurodivergent children, or coping with miscarriage, stillbirth, or the loss of a child often makes relationships more prone to strain and breakdown. Competition, envy, conflict, and difficulty in providing comfort and emotional regulation to each other because of the enormity of their own grief, despair, or stress can create a sense of loneliness and isolation that can be difficult to overcome without individual or relationship therapeutic support.

The journey to creativity, risk, and ambiguity

With such an eye-watering number of potential obstacles for the early adult, it is no wonder some seek therapy to help them find a path through the wilderness. Our work can be about helping the struggling young adult to become more psychologically and pragmatically settled, developing the mental, emotional, and practical strengths of adulthood: a strong sense of self-esteem, the ability to relate intimately, to communicate congruently, to take responsibility, and to take risks (Satir, 1988). It is about helping them become and feel like a man, woman, adult. We can examine with them their identity, values, beliefs, and choices, and help them explore, express, regulate, and become reconciled with painful feelings, disappointments, and intrapsychic, interpersonal and existential impasses. As energy is released and cathected, their greater potential for creativity and toleration of risk can help them experiment and learn to embrace excitement, joy, vitality, and uncertainty. They can learn to view life events and relationship in a more tolerant, open-minded manner, become aware of multiple truths, and accepting of the constraints and ambiguities of life: the successes and disappointments; grief and celebration; intimacy and autonomy; responsibility and fun; safety and risk; commitment and changeability; equilibrium and a sense of wonder. In doing so, they move from the adolescent world of fantasy, possibility, and hypothetical situations into the adult realms of realism, contradictions, compromise, and pragmatism (Labouvie-Vief, 2006). My client, Stan, had used therapy to explore his disappointment with adult life: his marriage, parenthood, and work. Growing in his ability to tolerate confliction and ambiguity, as well as the fears and joys of intimate connection, enabled him to make some changes whilst accepting the sacrifice of others. He wrote to me as we ended, still in the process of navigating early adulthood:

A while back I remember we talked about me becoming a man. I'm still working out what type of man I want to be but I feel I now have the security and confidence to properly find out. And hopefully grow into it. Which is a huge shift for me.

Therapy hadn't solved his problems, but had helped him take risks and explore creatively his commitments and identity. As the author, Virginia Woolf (1986), described, this move into adulthood was a birth of a sense of fellowship with other human beings as he took his place among them.

To help inspire our clients' creativity, I believe we need to be creative practitioners. We need to be inventive, imaginative, and welcome original thinking, ideas, and practices. And to do that, we need to be prepared to take risks, which can help demonstrate to our clients the concept of thoughtful risk-taking. Perhaps in no other life stage is this more important than for young adults, who have the potential to take great risks in carving out the sculpture of their lives. If we are not prepared to take risks with them, how will they be courageous and creative enough to risk venturing into the unknown, a prerequisite for learning and development? As Pablo Picasso, one of the boldest experimental and radical artists, is often attributed as saying: in doing that which we cannot do, we learn how to do it. We cannot move on in growth, development, identity or intimacy without risk – as a therapist or as an adult. Ackerman argues:

> Where there is no risk, the emotional terrain is flat and unyielding, and, despite all its dimensions, valleys, pinnacles, and detours, life will seem to have none of its magnificent geography, only a length. It began in mystery, and it will end in mystery, but what a savage and beautiful country lies in between.
>
> (Ackerman, 1991, p. 309)

The art and risk of both psychotherapy and the sculpting of adult life is paralleled in the creative arts. In a film by John Read (1961), Barbara Hepworth's description of sculpting could easily be describing psychotherapy with those in early adulthood:

> [becoming] lost in a world of space and creation with a thousand possibilities… which will carry one forward into unknown territory. The conclusion will be reached by a sense of balance. Suddenly before one's eyes is a new form … as one brings to it one's own special life.

Both therapist and client are at the same time sculptor, sculpture, and viewer. Through our own artistic eye on their lives, we invite early adults to have the eye of an artist to enable them to look more closely at the intricacies of their world: the dimensions, valleys, pinnacles, and detours of their life's terrain and their developing values, beliefs, and worldview. We encourage them to experiment with their identity and take risks with intimacy as they further sculpt the landscape of their adult life. We challenge them to accept that which is set in stone and that which can be sculpted further: to see and feel the intricacy of form, tone, colour, texture, energy, and rhythms of life and, in doing so, to discover their qualities, skills, beliefs, values, meanings, and desires. Therapy can help reveal their natural qualities and hidden energies in the same way that the sculptor reveals this in wood and stone. We do this by taking our own risks with relatedness. We communicate, implicitly and explicitly, our own expression of existence and what it is for us to be human, enabling them a glimpse of the unique sculpture of our own lives. And, in a beautiful gift of reciprocity and mutuality, the relationship invariably continues to sculpt our lives, too. In this way, we offer each other a reflection of our humanity that can bridge something of the universal chasm of loneliness and existential isolation.

Loneliness and isolation

Perhaps a deep-seated sense of loneliness, aloneness, or isolation is one of the most common and deeply painful challenges of early adulthood, experienced by many even when in loving relationships. Often, young adults have not yet understood the differentiation between being alone and being lonely; have not yet grasped that loneliness is an inevitable and passing feeling; or learned to tolerate different types of isolation. For some, isolation is viewed as an idyllic possibility for soul-searching and creativity; for others, as a punitive solitary confinement. Early adults may not yet have understood that it can be both, and perhaps have not yet discovered a comfort in their own company. As Albert Einstein reportedly described, living in solitude is painful in youth but delicious in the years of maturity (Schreiber, 1936). It can be helpful for us to consider three different but interrelated types of isolation (Yalom, 1980): Interpersonal, intrapsychic, and existential.

Interpersonal isolation

Interpersonal isolation is most commonly linked to loneliness in that it is an unwanted separation from others, a sadness and pain from being alone, and a feeling of lack or loss of companionship. It is experienced when a discrepancy exists between one's desired and one's actual level of social relationships, or, in other words, when we are not experiencing enough intimacy or connection. In his theory of psychobiological hungers, Eric Berne (1964, 1966) describes the innate need that human beings have to structure their time, with withdrawal at one end of the spectrum of time-structuring and intimacy at the other. In between are the relational modes of rituals, pastiming, activities, play (Cornell, 2015; Cowles-Boyd & Boyd, 1980), and games. Berne suggests that all modes, particularly psychological games, are inferior – and often defensive – alternatives to intimacy. I propose, however, that all can also offer connectedness and healthy routes into intimate relating (Cook, 2022). The problem arises when intimacy is desired but defended against through withdrawal or psychological games, and interpersonal isolation can be the consequence. To alleviate this, we need to learn to tolerate the tension between intimacy and withdrawal or isolation (Erikson, 1968); to practice stretching our muscles in our non-preferred modes of time-structuring; discover an understanding of the levels of intimacy and healthy withdrawal we personally benefit from and accepting how they might be different for others; and find our "kin" or "tribe" where we can feel more able to be authentic in relationship.

Loneliness and interpersonal isolation can be felt acutely for those in marginalised groups who have often experienced alienation throughout life and can find it particularly difficult to feel that their experience of life is being mirrored. One of my students, a single, gay man in early adulthood, faced a difficult dilemma between attending an important training weekend and going with his LGBTQ+ tribe to a contemporary performing arts festival. He described beautifully in a reflective piece, the dilemma of his choice and how he tolerated both polarities in finding a way – through healthy withdrawal from work and participating with loved ones in rituals, pastiming, activities, play, and intimacy – to alleviate his interpersonal isolation:

> I don't have children, nor am I getting pregnant, my friends are no longer getting married and I don't intend to get married. These are some of the reasons people miss training weekends. They are celebrations of a life that I will not be celebrating or be celebrated for. Getting together with the people I love most, my chosen family, for four days, having fun and sharing intimate and memorable moments is one of the ways I celebrate my life. And I have also found being with the [training] group, connecting and rupturing with them, to be the single most valuable element of my [transformation]. However, taking four days [off] work or study, enjoying the company of my nearest and dearest and soaking up the joyous environment of the festival, is what I need to recharge my tank. I find such energy and life in this pilgrimage and celebration, that it leaves me feeling full of love and life for weeks afterwards. I don't know if I have made the right decision, I hope I have.

Intrapsychic isolation

Intrapersonal or intrapsychic isolation is a form of self-alienation, "a process whereby one partitions off parts of oneself" (Yalom, 1980, p. 353) because of trauma, alienation, oppression, masking, or repetitive misattunements that have been left unrepaired. Transactional analysts may think of this type of intrapsychic isolation as different psychic levels of unhelpful introjected Parent and archaic Child ego states created through early experiences of isolation in relationship (Hargaden & Sills, 2002). Unacceptable and unbearable feelings and experiences are cut off from a person's true self, leaving devastating fragmentation or splitting of self, and embodied, nonverbal templates of relating that are often deeply unhelpful. Winnicott (1963) described this as the resourceful yet devastating hiding of the True Self – the "isolate" – in order to survive the unsurvivable. The resulting unbearable sense of intrapsychic isolation from the unique, authentic self, the source of creativity, growth, and power, is epitomised in his well-known phrase: "It is a joy to be hidden but a disaster not to be found" (Winnicott, 1965, p. 187). At its worst, it includes parts of self that have been "killed off" in a "soul murder", where radical isolation (Williams, 2022) is preferred to the terror and dread of human contact:

> The traumatic experiences that lead to the organisation of primitive defences belong to the threat to the isolated core, the threat of its being found, altered, communicated with. The defence consists in a further hiding of the secret self, even in the extreme to its projection and to its endless dissemination...
>
> (Winnicott, 1963, p. 187)

Williams talks about overcoming this self-isolation by respecting the person's need for privacy, attending to their overt personality whilst holding in mind their hidden authentic self: "There is an inherent tension between the needs of the authentic self and the needs of the evolving personality which, if attended to, builds a foundation for becoming a human being" (Williams, 2022, p. 10).

One of my creative supervisees describes intrapsychic isolation as the "holes and gaps" in life, memory, learning, and connection. She introduced me to the artist Barbara Hepworth, whose intentional holes and gaps in her sculptures were influenced by the holes and gaps in nature and are integral to the beauty and integrity of their form. Hepworth believed that holes and gaps enable a pure and gentle quality of light to pass through: a nut in its shell, a child in the womb, the structure of shells or crystals, bones in the human figure (Hepworth, 2012). Likewise, we can view the psychic holes and gaps as a window into a person's story and a means for light to get in.

Morag

Morag, a deeply sensitive, intuitive, and creative client in early adulthood, described feeling like she had huge gaps in her childhood and current experiences of living as an adult. She had few memories of her childhood and did not know how to be an adult in the world because she did not know who she was. She described how, as a child, she had found great solace in art and nature, and we gradually discovered together that they had provided her with much-needed security, connection, and escape from the pain, trauma, and isolation of abuse and neglect. One session she brought in a childhood scrapbook in which she had collected over many years postcards, pictures torn out of magazines, and sketches of famous pieces of art. In talking about what they had meant for her, we realised that in diverse ways, the artists had all expressed the primitive and spiritual forces of nature and humanity – the holes and gaps as well as the form; the peace and calm alongside the storm. Morag realised that by connecting with the artists' own inner striving for survival and growth that was communicated through their art, she had held on to threads of human connection that had alleviated her unbearable intrapsychic isolation and provided a protective and resilient shield for her own hidden isolate. She asked if we could meet outside in nature, and as we experienced the changing seasons together, we were able to talk about life, growth, death, and decay in a more creative way that was simultaneously connecting with the wounds of her early life as well as the adult she now was. The powerful combination of nature and human connection enabled Morag to come out of hiding and peer into her life's holes and gaps. She found meaning through the wonder of a hard-working ant colony forming a living bridge, the beauty of growing spring bulbs and decaying leaves, shiny conkers in a spiky defensive shell, the playfulness of dandelion clocks and leaping squirrels, a stunning shape-shifting starling murmuration. As she did so, she started creating a new scrapbook of artwork that depicted the natural world that we had shared and the form of her new adult landscape that she was sculpting. As her book gradually filled up, so did her adult life with new relationships, creative work opportunities, a home of her own, a greater toleration of her present losses and disappointments, and more colourful and artistic clothing that always had a nod to the natural world and expressed the beauty, vibrancy, and light and shade of life. Nature and art had held Morag through her original trauma in relationship, and it was the interrelatedness of nature, art, and human connection that enabled light to emerge through the shadowy holes and gaps of her intrapsychic isolation. Our creative relationship was helping her make meaning out of a life that had been previously sculpted for her, and begin to sculpt a different landscape for her present and future adult life.

Existential isolation

Art of all kinds can provide a bridge to transcend the third type of isolation: existential isolation. This underlies all other forms of isolation as it is universal to all humans and is present even in the midst of satisfying relationships with our tribe. It is a sense of being "inexorably alone… an unbridgeable gulf between oneself and any other being" (Yalom, 1980, p. 353) and "a separation between the individual and the world" (Yalom, 1980, p. 355). Nobody experiences existence and the world in exactly the same way as another because of our unique embodiment of existence, and thus "each of us is permanently separate from the other" (van Deurzen & Adams, 2011, p. 18).

Spinelli, however, argues that isolation and relatedness cannot be separated, and that "The self's experience of its own unique isolation is dependent upon the prior experience of relatedness" (Spinelli, 2015, p. 50). We were conceived and born in relation to another and are always "being-in-relation", interconnected with humanity, the environment, and the world we inhabit. Paradoxically, it is only because of our awareness of our relatedness to other humans that we have the ability to experience isolation from others and its associated sadness, despair, relief or joy (Spinelli, 2015, pp. 48–50). Even those withdrawing defensively from others because of fear of engulfment or profound self-alienation are tied to others in relationship because they need to be ever-vigilant to possible intrusion (Sartre, 1943/1956). Rather than seeing the tension between isolation and intimacy as being resolvable, as Erikson (1986) suggests, young adulthood can be about learning to tolerate the different polarities on a continuum and the ever-present paradoxical tension between them (van Deurzen, 2010). Like the solidity of form alongside gaps and holes, they are both intrinsic to the whole.

On holiday in Cornwall recently, the home of Hepworth for 30 years and a place where we had holidayed for 25 years since his birth, my son, his partner, and I experienced the most breath-taking and beautiful sunset from the beach, where the sky's magnificent streaks of blue, green, white, pink, red, orange, and gold could be seen in duplicate, reflected in the innumerable rockpools that had settled in the holes and gaps of undulations of sand. In sharing the almost painful and spiritual beauty, I had a profound sense of being deeply connected simultaneously to the landscape, my family, a higher spiritual force, and the past, present, and future of the universe. At the same time, I felt completely alone, realising that nobody in the world was experiencing exactly the same emotions, thoughts, and stirrings as I was, and acutely aware that one day I would be separated from this beautiful world and the people I love. This precious moment in time was fleeting, and as we left the glorious Cornish landscape and my son returned to his adult home, the depth of relatedness we had shared made the isolation of separation even more stark. Relatedness shines a light on isolation, and isolation reflects that light back on relatedness.

Heidi and James

Heidi and James, a married couple in their mid-30s with two young children, came to me for relationship therapy after Heidi's devastating discovery of James's affair. Both racked with guilt, despair, and pain, they described an unbearable loneliness in their marriage, an existential loneliness that can often feel worse in the presence of another than when physically alone. James felt isolated and suffocated with what felt like overwhelming responsibilities as a father, husband, and wage-earner in a job that stifled his creativity. He felt trapped by Heidi's emotional need for him and resented their increasingly obvious differences which left him feeling misunderstood and deadened: he was describing an interpersonal and intrapsychic isolation, and he wanted to combat it by finding his tribe and going out in the world to play, be creative, and grow. The woman he had connected with outside their marriage seemed to offer this connection and freedom, and temporarily alleviated some of his painful isolation.

Heidi, on the other hand, wanted to stay at home and nest with James and her children. She craved intimacy with James and, when he withdrew or rejected her advances, she felt hurt, resentful, and increasingly isolated at home alone with the children. The more James retreated, the more Heidi chased him, with James hurtfully accusing her of being too needy and demanding. We explored together their interlocking scripts and their "chase-withdrawal" dynamic, a vicious cycle whereby they both ended up hurt, resentful, and isolated. In doing so, we uncovered the intrapsychic isolation that both had experienced historically. Underlying Heidi's pressing need for intimacy was an archaic fear of abandonment, where, because of historical abandonment from the earliest months of life, she would feel the terror of exposure to what seemed like an unsurvivable existential aloneness. James feared engulfment and intrusion – a different form of abandonment – whereby he longed for intimacy but was terrified of it because of the threat to his isolate or core self. Both were terrified of their fundamental aloneness (Yalom, 1980), but each triggered this fear in the other.

As they faced this with courage and grieved the losses of their past, they learned to better identify their own and their partner's provocations. The intimacy, challenge, and feedback of the therapeutic relationship helped them to recognise their desires for and fears around intimacy, to interrupt unconscious enactments of past family relationships, and to practice being more intimate with me and each other.

Acknowledging our differences yet showing I could survive – and even enjoy – them, help them to begin appreciating their differences again rather than view them as an existential threat. Disclosure of some of my own relational struggles also reassured them that we all face similar tensions between intimacy and isolation. We discovered that James enjoyed and needed more time alone and less intimacy than Heidi, preferring to get his strokes (recognition or acknowledgement (Berne, 1964)) from activities and pastiming, whilst still craving some intimacy. Heidi particularly appreciated rituals and intimacy, whilst enjoying different activities from James. We explored creative and playful ways that they could manage their respective needs for intimacy and withdrawal and their differing desires for time-structuring, whilst holding firm and loving boundaries with each other. Communication improved, they became more creative at resolving conflict, and I felt like there were glimmers of hope. James was gradually learning to tolerate more intimacy and to communicate more effectively rather than withdrawing defensively, being clear when he needed healthy time alone. Heidi learned to better appreciate the intimacy that James offered rather than continually searching for more, and started looking to others to meet her intimacy needs that James could not. With the security of relatedness that the therapeutic relationship offered her, she also started feeling more able to practice being alone and looking to enjoy rather than be terrified of solitude. They both seemed to be accepting more the inevitable disappointment and sacrifice of relationships.

Yet fun and a life force in their relationship remained frustratingly elusive, and despite attempting to bring my vitality and humour into sessions in an attempt to stir theirs, there was a residual stuck feeling. Something was missing. Their relationship was painting by numbers rather than a spontaneous, creative, soulful work of art. Experimenting with a creative activity in an attempt to unlock the impasse, I invited them to sculpt in modelling clay an individual representation of what gave their lives meaning and how they wanted the landscape of their lives to look going forward. When they had finished, I invited them to compare the two models. A blanket of sadness and cold realisation descended on the room as they faced the striking starkness of their different landscapes. Life held different meanings for them, and they did not want the same thing for their futures. They were finally acknowledging irreconcilable differences; there were more holes and gaps than solid form. They both wept with grief as they started to accept that their relationship was ending.

It is 12 years since I last saw James and Heidi, and I have no idea whether, in retrospect, they are satisfied with or regret this important decision made in early adulthood. I imagine there will be elements of both. To paraphrase Kierkegaard: "If you divorce, you will regret it; if you do not divorce, you will also regret it". Staying together takes risk; sometimes ending involves even greater risk. Courage and creativity would have been necessary to stay together, and courage and creativity were needed to change radically the landscape of their adult lives. With the multitude of possibilities open to them, early adults are continually travelling through an unknown, uncertain, savage, and beautiful landscape that is being creatively sculpted with every choice or imposition. Young adults need to know that they can take risks, make mistakes, and survive them, learn from them, and grow from them. They need to experience that even gaps and holes help to form the contours, valleys, and pinnacles of their life, and to appreciate the light that shines through them to enable creativity from destruction and a future that has potential for survival, growth, integrity, and forgiveness. I hope Heidi and James have been able to find this. It is the transcendent art of relationship, the art of a relational and existential psychotherapy, and the art of spiritual and creative endeavours that offer possibilities for the creation of a new landscape out of destruction and isolation.

Chapter 9

Middle adulthood

Re-visiting our dreams

One of my favourite walks is around the stunningly beautiful Cwm Pennant in Eryri (Snowdonia). I discovered it in midlife when returning to North Wales with my young adult sons, retracing the steps of the happy family caravan holidays of my youth. A poem by Eifion Wyn (cited in Cymdeithas Eryri Snowdonia Society, 2018) of the same name inspired me to seek out 'Cwm Pennant': roughly translated, his final soul-stirring lines cried out: "Why, Lord, did you make Cwm Pennant so beautiful, when a shepherd's life is so short?". As I walked alone through the awe-inspiring valley, I felt the touch of the "Sacred Present" (Carlsen, 1988, p. 241, citing Alfred North Whitehead). The vivid sights, sounds, and smells of majestic mountains, glimmering brooks, abandoned shepherds' huts, and disused quarry railway, evoked for me the almost seamless merging of past, present, and future: the people that had walked and worked in this magnificent valley for thousands of years, the long-dead poet, my original family, my sons, and their potential children's children who I hoped might walk amongst the same mountains when I am no longer alive to enjoy them. In that moment I could understand the homesickness, yearning and nostalgia for Wales that the Welsh call "hiraeth" (from "hir", meaning "long", and "aeth", meaning "sorrow or grief"). As has become increasingly familiar for me in middle age, I felt simultaneously a strong appreciation for my past; a yearning in my soul for my lost childhood; a comfort in being "home"; a humility, gratitude, and awe at the beauty and majesty that transcended the tiny speck of my humanity; and a grief that I cannot hold on to this beauty forever.

For many in middle adulthood, this combination of grief, nostalgia, longing, regret, and urgency are common as we wake up to the reality of our own mortality. We see less life ahead of us than behind us and time becomes more figural: anxiety about time running out, a longing to go back in time, regrets about time spent, a desire to make up for lost time, fears about the time ahead, despair that we will one day finally run out of time, an urgency to make the

DOI: 10.4324/9781003475217-12

most of remaining time. The philosopher-singer-songwriter, David Bowie, spoke about the tensions of "Time" in the 2022 film about his life, *Moonage Daydream* by Brett Morgen:

> Time... It's something that straddles past and future without ever quite being present... there's a tension of a most unfathomable nature...You're aware of a deeper existence, maybe a temporary reassurance that indeed there is no beginning, no end... a deep and formidable mystery. All is transient, does it matter?

The search for meaning

The transition into "Middle life" (Jung, 1931/1970) or "Middle age" (Neugarten, 1968) often brings with it this sense of meaninglessness in existence and a striving to create some order, purpose, and meaning from our struggles (Frankl, 1946/1969). The growing awareness of limited time and a myriad of changing and often challenging life circumstances can make some experience a sense of disorientation (Gollnick, 2008); a grief and anxiety as we experience the death of aspects of our old self; and a spiritual development as we re-evaluate life (Gubi, 2015), particularly for those who are psychologically minded, "unconventional", and who have experienced adversity in their lives (Wink & Dillon, 2002). The resulting existential anxiety can lead them to ask themselves about their lives, "Is this really it?", which Elliot Jaques (1965) described as the "mid-life crisis".

The mid-life crisis

The life crisis of middle adulthood can sometimes involve drastic and sudden changes made to marriages, relationships, careers, goals, identity, or creative endeavours in an avid or desperate search for meaning, vitality, and generativity (Erikson, 1968). The stereotypical image is that of the middle-aged person who abdicates responsibilities and drives away from family and work in an open-topped sports car with a new partner 20 years younger in an attempt to re-live their youth. Some defend against death, ageing, and the givens of human existence in this way, but for others a life crisis (at any stage of life) is about an excruciating period of crisis depression (Kegan, 1982) as they face head on the many and various challenges of this life stage, and the associated meaninglessness, regrets, monotony, or finality of life. Levinson (1978, 1996) suggested that this inner turmoil can also involve slow and steady change rather than extreme life adjustments. Whichever way it is experienced, the unbearable pain of crisis or ontological insecurity (Laing, 1960) can make middle adults feel exposed, vulnerable, and without a solid identity.

Nicole and Rosie

My own mid-life crisis hit devastatingly in my early forties when my husband of 20 years left me very unexpectedly and painfully. Having been together since our teens, being alone and a single parent felt terrifying, threatening my whole existence and identity. The foundations of life gave way as I disappeared into a dark, cavernous sink hole of anxiety, despair, and crisis depression. I would wake in the night in an anxious panic, gripped with terror of death, aloneness, and my non-being. I was sustained by the support of my family, friends, therapist, supervisor, and cat companions, who helped me gradually find a new identity and grow through the devastation. Two clients – Nicole and Rosie – who had both been left suddenly by their husbands for other women, were also unaware companions on my crisis journey. They shared similar stories of devastation, rejection, betrayal, the shattering of trust, and hopes and expectations for the future, a sense of injustice, profound grief, the disorientation of their past "truth" now feeling like a lie, and the sense of dread that bad things could happen at any time. I did not explicitly disclose our similarities, but both women later told me that they had always known implicitly that I had also navigated similar pain and crisis. I think this is because I had gone to my inner depths through my own experiences, which enabled me to offer my authentic presence, vulnerability as well as strength, the courage to challenge as well as support, and involvement in truly going with them into their pain. This invited them into the vulnerability and intimacy of sharing their raw and honest struggle. As van Deurzen suggests:

> The person who is at the rock bottom of existence and who has nothing more to lose will instantly sniff out any form of patronizing or missionary zeal or, indeed, of fakery and pretence. Only the therapist who has faced their personal depth of self will be able to make a difference for the person so utterly lost at the edge or, worse, in the depth of the abyss.
>
> (Van Deurzen 2012, pp. 198–199)

Kegan describes it as offering "a most intimate and usually unexpected companionship – not as another object in the world, but as a fellow hanger-in-the-balance" (Kegan, 1999, pp. 275–276). Without imposing onto them my personal experiences or "truth", I always endeavour to speak truthfully from my soul: as Farber suggests, "Speaking truthfully is a more fitting ambition than speaking the truth" (Farber, 2000, p. 10). Truthful speaking helps them see that I have moved from breakdown into breakthrough (Laing, 1960), from the dark wood into a lighter clearing of greater meaning, creativity, and vitality, but also that I, too, sometimes re-visit the dark wood – or discover another forest. With this honesty, I offer hope, kinship, challenge, and inspiration, which they also offer me. We are "co-facilitators of re-balancing".

Spiritual re-balancing

Nicole's spiritual quest also mirrored mine. Just as my own life crisis had, her devastation had shaken her previously sustaining Christian faith, and speaking about it with her reignited my own spiritual angst. Feeling somewhat of a spiritual void and even some judgement about faith in my psychotherapy community (which is thankfully now starting to shift), I sought the help of a "spiritual accompanier" – a multi-denominational "soul friend" and companion on my spiritual journey. Putting aside her own beliefs, she helped me grapple with my tensions, disappointments, and fears, investigating what I wanted my spiritual beliefs to be now as a middle-aged adult rather than what I had swallowed whole as a child and adolescent. Most importantly for me, I became more comfortable with simply not knowing. As I shifted and tolerated better the uncertainty of life, death, and faith, so did Nicole. This was shown to me in a dream, which I recount as if experiencing it in the present:

> Nicole arrives for her session and I realise that I have left a dead body in my therapy room. I speak with Nicole about it and we decide we are happy to leave it there. We move on to talk about other things, occasionally smiling as we glance over to the body and acknowledge its presence, then carry on contentedly with our previous conversation.

The contrast was striking between my anxiety-ridden, isolating death nightmares at the height of my crisis and the companionship and acceptance of death in this dream. Death was in the room and it was okay. I decided to share my dream with Nicole to invite explicit dialogue about her feelings about death; like spirituality, death is so often avoided in therapy, which does our clients a great disservice. Over time, this helped her face at greater depth the death of her old self, the current discombobulating void, and her feelings about how she wanted to live more fully her remaining new life. Kegan describes this reconfiguration of meaning-making:

> the dying of a way to know the world which no longer works, a loss of an old coherence with no new coherence immediately present to take its place. And yet a new balance again and again does emerge. … Still, it is a *new* life, not a return or a recovery.
>
> (Kegan, 1999, p. 266)

Life after a crisis is never the same; aspects of the person that they were have died, but a new self will emerge. There will still be moments of pain, isolation, and angst in the dark wood, but there will be more times in the bright clearing of joy, connection, intimacy, and meaning. This is the same for every person in middle adulthood: they are not the same person as they were in youth and they need to discover new meaning and the person they are now in this life stage.

The challenges of middle adulthood

Facing death and decline

There are many reasons why those in middle adulthood are more prone to existential crisis. Decline starts becoming more obvious, and with it, a fear of ageing, old age, and death: a less youthful body shape and strength, wrinkles, vision deterioration, menopausal symptoms, prostate difficulties, challenges with sexual arousal or erectile dysfunction, bodily aches and pains, memory changes, ageism. It may also be the first time that a person has come face-to-face with death, a near-death experience, or a felt threat to existence through bereavement, relationship breakdown, redundancy, serious illness, or accident. They may witness these situations occurring for a growing number of loved ones, and be confronted with the reality that "this could be me".

The sandwich generation

Middle adulthood has also been dubbed the "sandwich generation" (Miller, 1981), squeezed between work, elderly parents, and children or grandchildren. Particularly in individualistic societies where responsibilities are not so readily shared by extended family and community, women can feel quite isolated carrying much of the mental or practical load for caring, often at the same time as facing the transition into menopause. Women in midlife are also particularly likely to face economic, social, and employment disadvantage (Berk, 2023). Men still often feel a cultural responsibility for being the "breadwinner", which can make facing retirement or redundancy particularly stressful. Caring for elderly parents (particularly if living with them) can lead to overwhelm, conflict, relationship difficulties, depression, and emotional, physical, and financial stress. This can be particularly acute if also struggling with their children's turbulent adolescence. Being faced with parents' ageing can also lead to greater levels of anxiety about their own old age and death.

Children leaving home or finding partners during one's middle adulthood can bring a sense of joy, pride, and freedom, but also grief and a void if parenthood has been the person's main purpose in life. If they stay living at home, or return as emerging adults, this can bring its own challenges around independence, values, and responsibility as new parent-adult relationships are negotiated. The middle generation often have an urge to be "kinkeeper" – the family "glue" who brings everyone together – which can be rewarding but also disappointing and saddening if the family is not as hoped for because of divorce, death, or relational difficulties. This role can be fulfilled by becoming grandparents, which many enjoy for the fun and companionship without the child-rearing responsibilities, but increasingly grandparents are taking on child-caring roles to help their children with work and finances. This has the reward of deeper relationships with their grandchildren, but it can also be exhausting and pressurising, particularly if there are differences in opinions about their care. Becoming a grandparent can stir existential angst about ageing and passing on the baton, whilst not becoming grandparents can be a big life disappointment and may stir previous losses or regrets for those who did not have children.

Work and relationships

All of these changes may put pressure on marriages and long-term partnerships in middle life as the couple seek new meaning, navigate the "empty nest", and move in different directions with work, hobbies, and friendships. People tend to have fewer friendships in middle life as they grow more aware of the preciousness of time, but women in particular increasingly protect those of value (Berk, 2023). For those who have left long-term relationships or who have been single for some time there can be fears about growing old alone, and it can be both intimidating and exciting to face the virtual and real-life dating scene. Men in middle life often move more quickly than women into new romantic relationships, frequently having a new relationship to go to before ending the existing one (Levitt & Cici-Gokaltun, 2011). New partners in middle adulthood are often at different life stages, may still be recovering from divorce or the death of a previous partner, and may involve conflicts over step-children, the blending of two families, or whether to have children together.

Those in middle adulthood are often at the peak of their career, providing meaning, status, and fulfilment. But with increased responsibilities, and after a long demanding career, there is also a risk of burnout. There can be the risk of redundancy in an age-focused society, particularly with the rise of young blood and Artificial Intelligence. Retirement planning can lead to a sense of freedom and excitement, but also anxiety over loss of status, finances and purpose. For those who have been raising children or in mundane or unfulfilling jobs, the realisation that it is "now or never" can lead to a radical change in career, which can be both enlivening and terrifying.

Generativity versus stagnation

With challenge and crisis, however, comes opportunity for transformation. The word "crisis" in Chinese is represented by the characters for "danger" and "opportunity" (Kegan, 1999), and Jung suggested that facing death in the second half of life can give motivation to make the most of living: to "discover in death a goal towards which one can strive" (Jung, 1931/1970, p. 402). Having goals keeps people generative and prevents stagnation; Kierkegaard (cited in van Deurzen, 2012, p. 197) even suggested that victory is man's greatest enemy as it alienates him from himself. The "jolts" of life can shift us out of any middle life stagnation or alienation into more creative, generative, and innovative ways of thinking, feeling, being, and meaning-making. Often, the greater the existential angst, the more profound the change or the work of art. It was the existential longings and grief of "hiraeth" arising from cultural oppression, for example, which led to the Welsh fight to reclaim their heritage, traditions, and language.

Erikson (1968) suggested that successful middle adulthood was about navigating this tension between generativity and stagnation. Of course, this is culturally and socially determined. In Japan, for example, middle age is viewed as an extended period of socially recognised, productive maturity (Menon, 2015), whilst menopause is celebrated by the indigenous Māori in New Zealand as a transition into spiritual eldership. In other Western cultures, however, the menopause can still be ridiculed or ignored, and women are still rated as less attractive and having more negative personality characteristics than middle-aged men, despite many reporting feeling more assertive, confident, and capable of resolving life's problems (Lemish & Muhlbauer, 2012). For those with significant financial hardship and lower socio-economic status, middle age may also be more focused on survival than generativity.

It can be helpful for us to confront ageist and sexist stereotypes and affirm middle adults in their power, skills, and gained wisdom. Research shows that middle adults can be particularly skilled at identifying the positives in difficult situations, anticipating and planning ways to handle future discomforts, and using humour to express ideas and feelings without offending others (Diehl, Coyle, & Labouvie-Vief, 1996). Often at the peak of their careers or with extensive experience of family relationships, they are also often talented at applying their knowledge, intuition, and problem-solving skills. Opportunities for increased responsibilities, leadership positions, and status at work and in the community can lead to a greater sense of life satisfaction, self-acceptance, personal power, autonomy, and environmental mastery (Berk, 2023) and can help them feel they are closer to fulfilling their potential. With a positive mind-set and the satisfaction of generativity, it is possible for middle adults to feel like they are in the "prime of life".

Passing on the torch

With generativity comes a growing capacity for the virtues of love, care, and wisdom (Erikson, 1968) and a desire to give to humanity, repair the world, and enrich the lives of others. There is a movement from focusing on self and self-expression to "passing on the torch" to future generations (Vaillant, 2002), potentially satisfying an evolutionary urge to make a contribution that will survive our death and to protect the future by offering inspiration and a stabilising force to the radical new ideas of younger adults. Gubi (2015) describes middle adulthood as the time for finding a balance between the spiritual outward turn of the self towards the world, and an inward spiritual focus on order, coherence, meaning, and purpose. Family, mentoring, teaching, therapy, supervision, coaching, community service, communication of ideas, creating products or works of art, scientific discoveries, and political or social activation are all ways that the middle adult can be generative. It is undoubtedly a mutually beneficial relational process, with both learning from each other and enabling the more experienced adult to feel fulfilled and needed. Transactional Analysis' (TA's) focus on the "pathology" of rescuing can sometimes discount our existential need to be needed; Angyal argues:

> we ourselves want to be needed. We not only have needs, we are also strongly motivated by *neededness*. To be of no use to anything or anybody would make life intolerable... we are restless when we are not needed, because we feel "unfinished", "incomplete", and we can only get completed in and through these relationships.
>
> (Angyal, 1965, p. 20)

Power and vulnerability

Being needed and purposeful can help the middle adult feel greater power-from-within. Power is an ever-present, ever-changing existential certainty in every relationship and in all aspects of our lives. It can be used for good or ill; the aim is therefore not to remove or deny power but to minimise domination and maximise healthy assertion, resistance, generativity, and mutual recognition. Hoogendijk (1988) says that humans always balance on the polarity of power and impotence, wanting to affirm their power yet constantly finding themselves vulnerable. This balance can shift in middle adulthood: feeling a sense of power in being successful in their career or positions of responsibility, and/or a sense of declining power in terms of physical or cognitive capabilities; decreasing influence on adult children; or the powerlessness of illness, relational breakdown, redundancy, or retirement. Such experiences can confront harshly a sense of "specialness and personal inviolability" (Yalom, 1980) that had previously protected them against their death anxiety. Alternatively, like my client, Nicole, their lack of control over difficult circumstances might challenge their notion of a supernatural "Ultimate Rescuer" (Yalom, 1980). Without these defences, their sense of power can be shattered, facing instead the powerlessness and vulnerability of their mortality and the fragility of life. Levinson (1978) suggests that the resolution of existential tensions is the work of middle age: young-old, destruction-creation, masculinity-femininity, and engagement-separateness. True power is balancing both polarities, and living with vitality despite knowing we will fall down and ultimately face inevitable death (Tillich, 1954).

Mutuality and collaboration

Generativity involves a shift from self-interest into generosity, and from competitive attempts at domination and control to the courage of cooperation and collaboration (Sartre, 1946/2007). This movement from power-over to power-with (Proctor, 2017) must involve the humility of acknowledging our vulnerability and need for the other.

> To be generous with what we have is the key to good human relations. As we give away, so we feel more in tune with what we really are, that is, nothing. As we become emptied, we become ready to receive in return. When, in mutuality, we give to each other we never run out of what we need.
>
> (Van Deurzen & Iacovou, 2013, p. 5)

As fellow "hangers-in-the-balance", existential therapists respect the asymmetry of our position (Aron, 1996) whilst aiming for collaboration and mutuality in the demonstration of generosity, vulnerability, humility, and the ability to receive as well as give. In this way, role and social power can be transcended by a felt sense of equality in our common humanity (Brink, 1987). Yet power can only be genuinely shared when each individual has a sense of their inherent value and "power-from-within". The social and historical power and powerlessness of both client and therapist will affect how they perceive their capability to have power in the relationship and how they view the dyad's sharing of power. Much will also depend on each of their current sense of power in their respective stage of life. Frantz Fanon, the French Afro-Caribbean psychiatrist and political-philosopher, argued that we should simply aim to touch the other:

"Superiority? Inferiority? Why not the simple attempt to touch the other, to feel the other, to explain the other to myself?" (Fanon, 1952/2008, p. 231). This is the power-with of phenomenological dialogue: "the conscious movement of the therapist towards the other as an ethical stance allows true dialogue of unequals, in which both therapist and client are powerful *and* non-powerful" (Larner, 1999, p. 48).

Discovering new values and beliefs

Dialogue can help the middle adult get to know the essence of who they are in this new life stage, exploring their spiritual dimension of life, making meaning and connecting to something greater than ourselves. Underpinning this is our value system: what we live for and might be willing to die for. This might be family, religion, creative pursuits; exploration; caring for others, animals, or the environment; sporting or academic achievements; work or vocation; philosophical or political ideology; fighting for justice. Difficulties can emerge in middle adulthood when we want to relinquish or change old values that have silently, powerfully, and perhaps non-consciously been our life guide to this point. Particularly for those with a rigid belief system, it can be hard to accept that our values about the world, life, or what is beyond are never fixed and are always open to change. Heidegger (1927/2010) suggests that we are helping clients search for an "openness to being", where truth is ever-changing, never completed, and revealed dynamically over time. Carlsen describes this as "movement from the dark wood to new understandings, new experiences, and new meanings" (Carlsen, 1988, p. 3). But movement into the light from the familiar dark wood can be blinding and painful. In 2010, 33 Chilean miners who had been trapped underground for 69 days were brought to the earth's surface wearing specialised sunglasses to protect their adapting retinas from being damaged by the daylight. The discovery and re-evaluation of our beliefs and value system in middle adulthood can be like re-emerging into the sunlight after years in a cave. It can be comforting and relieving, bringing direction and purpose to our lives, whilst also disturbing and uprooting to our identity and sense of self if we are considering changing that which has been handed down to us by our families and cultures. Life can feel "absurd" or meaninglessness when we realise that we are the only one who defines our beliefs, and the enormity of the freedom and responsibility for our change can evoke existential anxiety. Discovering the therapist's different value system can sometimes be the confrontation our clients need to discover that difference can be manageable.

Meaning and meaninglessness

Spinelli (2015) argues that rigidity, either/or thinking, and fundamentalism can result from an obsessive search for meaning, where we reject, denigrate, or deny the value or existence of something that does not fit with our view of meaning. To guard against this, he says we must also accept the disturbance of meaning-lessness. As a school teacher, I took a group of 15-year-old students on a his-tory trip to Berlin, where we visited a Nazi concentration camp. After their shocking and horrifying experience of fundamentalism at its worst, some were affronted that I organised a bowling excursion that evening, disorientated by the juxtaposition of "meaningless" fun after such profound disturbance. At the end of the evening, a deeply thoughtful student came to thank me. "I thought I shouldn't have fun after experiencing what we did today. It all feels so point-less. But then I thought of all the fun those people had missed out on. So, I felt like I should make sure I have pointless fun while I can". The shock to her frame of reference helped her to re-evaluate her value system, acknowledging both the meaning and meaninglessness in fun and the horrific meaninglessness of genocide.

It is often "the shock of the new" (Hughes, 1991) of meaninglessness that enables new creativity, discovery, playfulness, and imagination in meaning-making. The artist, Tracey Emin, was popularly lambasted in the 1990s for her controversial and evocative autobiographical and confessional artwork. She was particularly criticised by art critics for the "sensationalist" and "solipsis-tic" installation, "*My Bed*" (1998), which featured empty vodka bottles, used condoms, and blood-stained underwear in an exhibition of a depressive four days in her life. It was described by some as "meaningless", yet it sold for over £2.5 million in 2014, and Emin was honoured as one of the first female profes-sors at the Royal Academy and made a Dame for services to British art. After the "meaningless" shock of the new, meaning was found in her honesty, vulner-ability, feminism, confrontation to the stigma of mental health, and the wider questioning of the personal meaning, vitality, and value of art as a communi-cation and transcendence of humanity. As Emin herself reflected in an inter-view on the "South Bank Show" in 2001, it was her humanity that gave her seemingly meaningless work meaning: "I realised that I was much better than anything I had ever made... I then realised I was the work, I was the essence of my work."

The power of dreaming

It is our humanity that is the essence of our work as therapists. And our ther-apy is our own personal and individual artwork that communicates our unique humanity. Our clients can be impacted by our humanity in the same way that we can be impacted by the artist's, author's, musician's or actor's expression of shared humanity in art, books, music, films, theatre. We can also discover our humanity in the creative expression of fantasies, daydreams, and dreams. Dreams – waking or sleeping – are a creative way we think, feel, hope, imagine, resolve tensions, make meaning, and rewrite our existence and our future. When faced with the limits of our existence in middle adulthood, listening to these dreams can help us find new ways to live with vitality and passion. Existentialists believe that these are as important as our waking "real-life" experiences, thoughts and feelings. Rather than trying to interpret the unconscious symbolism or wish fulfilment of dreams (Freud, 1900/1953), Medard Boss (1977, influenced by Heidegger, 1927/2010) advocated a thorough phenomenological investigation of the dream, helping the client describe and clarify the content from different angles as if it was a waking-world event. The client can then find their own meaning to shine a light on their waking world and create new possibilities for living and managing their existential tensions.

Kerr

Kerr, a 44-year-old Scottish gay man, described feeling stuck, unfulfilled, and restless in his work and marriage, yet he was scared of making any significant life-changing decisions. A disturbing dream he shared at the beginning of our relationship proved to be the catalyst for Kerr to open up to his existential struggles. Asking him to repeat it in the present-tense helped Kerr to re-live the dream as if it was happening in waking life:

> I am driving up to a crossroads and am shocked to see my husband lying in the middle of the road. He has just been hit by a car and looks dead. The driver of the car is ringing for the ambulance and a woman is giving him CPR. I am hesitant to stop; it's an unsafe junction, my husband is being cared for, and I want to get home away from the trauma. I suddenly see my colleague, Joe, in a colourful car driving towards my husband's body. I keep driving towards my home and hope Joe follows me. When he sees the body he drives really fast away from it, in the opposite direction to me. I am disappointed. I feel guilty for leaving my husband but relieved he is being looked after and that I'm not involved. My brother comes to see me later. He was in the car with Joe. He says, "don't worry, he'll be back, he was scared but he likes you". I feel warm and excited.

Over many months we returned again and again to the dream, exploring it from alternative perspectives, and focusing at different times on the people, the feelings, the events, and how Kerr thought they might be linked to his past, present, and future. It is the multiple possible meanings of the dream that make them so powerful, and new significance can be discovered at each re-telling. I asked him what the three men in the dream meant to him: his husband, colleague, and brother. He described his past relationships with men and the powerlessness he had felt as the youngest of four dominant boys and the only gay member of the family, when his vulnerability was not appreciated or respected. Asking him how he saw vulnerability in his dream, he realised he had driven away from his husband in his time of need. "I just didn't want to get involved", he admitted. "How do you feel that you chose not to be involved?" I asked. "Guilty but relieved", he replied, then, after a period of silence, he added, "I think that's how I feel about our distance in real life, too". This revelation enabled us to explore the conflict Kerr felt between guilt and relief when he considered ending the relationship. We investigated the values instilled in him from his Catholic background that marriage was for life, alongside the tension of messages about gay marriage being "sinful". Having previously reconfigured his belief system about gay marriage, he found it painful to consider re-evaluating his values about divorce, describing feeling stuck between a rock and a hard place and not knowing which direction to turn. I reminded him about the crossroads in his dream and asked him what sense he made of it. He half-laughed. "It feels obvious now... I'm at a crossroads in my life. No wonder I'm stuck, there are four different possible directions!" I playfully confronted him, "Five actually. You could stay in the middle with the dead body". Kerr shuddered. "I can't even bear to think about that". We explored his repulsion, with Kerr making links with the stagnancy of staying in a "dead" relationship and job. Enquiring about his relief at leaving the scene of the accident he began to realise his fears of being out of control and not being able to stop bad things happening in life, leaving him reluctant to initiate change.

Kerr was resistant to contemplating his own death, so I turned again to his more accessible dream. I asked him about the significance of his colleague Joe and his speeding away from the dead body. His response was the polar opposite of the deadness he felt in his work and marriage. "I feel alive and powerful when I'm with Joe," he said. "It's like life speeds up and becomes more colourful – I guess like his car!". Van Deurzen (2012) suggests that when we are open to something new, we find them in our dreams. Dreams can therefore be an expression of a growing physis or erotic vitality, new possibilities, a desire for growth and a realisation of what is holding us back. Through phenomenological investigation of his dream, Kerr was realising that Joe was bringing back to life his passion, powerfulness, aliveness, sexuality, desire. Kerr's dream was giving him new motivation to move from death into life by choosing a different life direction.

Yet Kerr was in conflict because Joe was in a junior position to him at work and he felt very aware of not misusing his role power. I asked him what sense he made of his brother's reassurance in the dream. He talked about how he was closest to his brother out of all his family, admiring and often submissive as the younger sibling, but sharing a loving, trusting relationship. "So, power and love together", I clarified, "that's quite a potent combination". Tillich (1954) suggests that both love and power are ways of approaching the other in an attempt to overcome separateness and difference; if power is full of love it can seek assertive union rather than destruction. Kerr saw that love and power were a part of his relationship with Joe as well as his brother, and we discussed different types of power. He decided that he needed to let Joe drive away to empower him to decide whether he wanted to drive back to the love and union that Kerr could offer him. "What about your relationship with your husband?", I asked, my enquiry unintentionally but inevitably bringing my own value system into our relationship. "Are you judging me?", Kerr confronted. I spoke truthfully, disclosing that my present value system was to end with one monogamous relationship before embarking on another, but that Kerr needed to decide for himself what his beliefs were, and whether he wanted to keep or change his existing values about relationships. The intrapsychic and interpersonal tussle brought an energy and healthy aggression to our relating, which eventually proved to be the impetus Kerr needed to make change. He decided that he couldn't go back to the destruction of the dead body, and started moves to change his career and leave his husband. Our inquiry into his dream and our relationship was helping him find the courage to individualise, affirm his own identity and power, and choose his own reconfigured value system that enabled him to go in the direction of life and love rather than death.

In our final session, Kerr told me about a dream he had had the night before.

I am out walking with Joe. I am self-conscious that our colleagues are nearby, and I feel some shame that we are together. He puts his arm round me, and our colleagues look up. I'm surprised that they're not bothered; they turn back to what they were doing and we walk on uninterrupted. My shame goes. I snuggle into his chest and we give each other a tender kiss and smile at each other. I feel warm, loving and comforted.

"You sound a lot calmer than in your first dream," I noticed. "Yes, I didn't want to wake up from this dream," he smiled, "I just hope my dreams are writing real life". Whether Kerr fulfilled his dream with Joe, or with another man that he was perhaps yet to meet, I have no doubt that his dreams were helping him write the next chapter of his ever-evolving life story of love, power and generativity. As Van Deurzen suggests: "Designing one's dreams as blueprints for reality is the beginning of a life which brings fulfilment" (Van Deurzen, 2012, p. 180).

Middle adulthood can be a time for re-visiting our dreams and looking at them anew. Like re-reading a book or seeing a film or piece of art again, re-visiting a significant dream will speak to us in a new and relevant way that perhaps we were not previously open to hearing or seeing. Through dreams, art, and therapy, we can gain an understanding of our existence and find meaning in our humanity, enabling us to see the sometimes-harsh realities of existence from a safe distance. Perhaps no time in life is this more important than in tempestuous middle adulthood. In his book, "Voyage en Italie" (that inspired the French artist, Paul Cézanne), art theorist Hippolyte Taine describes the use of art in a way that could easily be applied to both dreaming and therapy:

In open country I would rather meet a sheep than a lion; but behind the bars of a cage, I would rather see a lion than a sheep. Art [therapy, dreams] is exactly that sort of cage; by removing the terror, it preserves interest. Hence, safely and painlessly, we may contemplate the glorious passions, the heartbreaks, the titanic struggles, all the sound and fury of human nature elevated by remorseless battles and unrestrained desires. And surely, then it has the power to move and to stir.

(Taine, 1864, cited in Krook, 2021)

Chapter 10

Mature adulthood
Living well, laughing often, and loving much

"A family with an old person has a living treasure of gold" asserts an ancient Chinese proverb, while Oscar Wilde (in "The Picture of Dorian Gray" saves his respect for the young: "It's absurd to talk of the ignorance of youth. The only people to whose opinions I listen now with any respect are people much younger than myself. They seem in front of me. Life has revealed to them her latest wonder" (Wilde, 1891/1913, p. 239). In contrast, Ancient Israel's King Solomon, renowned for his wisdom in old age, is somewhat more measured about age, pronouncing that "The glory of the young is their strength; the grey hair of experience is the splendour of the old" (Proverbs 20:29, New Living Translation, 1996). Currently sitting in the midlife no-man's-land between youth and old age (feeling neither old nor young), I often do not see chronological age as significant, but can benefit from the wisdom, strength, empathy, and experience of mature adults whatever their actual age. I was recently deeply touched and humbled by the kindness of my local community of neighbours – of mixed ages but all with a maturity borne through adversity – who offered their time, strength, and experience in supporting me when my beloved cat was killed by a car outside my home. It was the mature adults who had experienced their own struggle with trauma and bereavement (of both animal and human companions) who knew what I needed: they were the strangers who stopped their cars in an attempt to help my cat and find her owner; my next-door-neighbour, widowed as a young adult, who wrapped her body in a beautiful embroidered piece of cloth and took her into her house, then empathically told me of her death when I returned home; the newly widowed friend two doors away who came to offer me her companionship. Yet equally supportive and sensitive was her son in early adulthood – my son's best friend who had recently lost his father after a devastating illness – who, in the absence of my own sons, dug a grave in my garden and helped me bury my feline companion. The comfort, kindness, and wisdom of these mature adults, who had known far greater adversity than my current one, was truly humbling and sustaining.

We all need role models who have navigated well the transition into the life stage we are currently facing, and those who have embraced older age can be

DOI: 10.4324/9781003475217-13

particularly inspiring. In turning to write about life stages that I have not yet lived, it is my aim and hope that I can do so with a level of humility, awareness of my ignorance and naivety, and a willingness to learn. For these are some of the most important characteristics of the mature adult. As my transition into mature adulthood comes closer, I am inspired by those I have observed who are steering effectively this course: my parents, siblings, clients, students, supervisees, therapist, supervisors, colleagues, authors. These mature adults have the humility to recognise how much they do not know; the enthusiasm to keep learning from those of any age or level of experience; the self-belief to recognise their wealth of knowledge, experience, and wisdom; and the love and passion to pass this on to others. They prove that mature adulthood can be a productive, innovative, and growthful period of life. Far from the now outdated view that older age is a time for disengagement from activity and preoccupation on the past in anticipation of death (Cumming and Henry's (1961) social disengagement theory), successful ageing involves the overcoming of difficulties with resilience, humility, and optimism, and an involvement in life that gives potential for vitality, maturity and regeneration (Levin-Landheer, 1982; Havighurst's (1972) "activity theory"). The definition of old age is also changing; where once it was seen to begin in someone's 60s in Western societies (Erikson, 1968; Havighurst, 1972; Levinson, 1986) – and still is in many areas of the world (World Health Organization, 2024) – the global shift in population ageing through better living standards and advances in medical treatment has highlighted significant differences between the active, healthy, and productive "Young-old" and the declining, increasingly dependent "Old-old" (Neugarten, 1968) that are not determined solely by chronological age. To account for the very different ways that people experience older age, I have therefore divided the later life stages into "Mature adulthood" (Havighurst's (1972) "Maturity") and "Late adulthood".

Inspiration of mature adulthood

With favourable life circumstances, optimism, and strong will, mature adulthood can be extended well into old age; some people may live into their 90s and never reach late adulthood. At 90, my mother needs care because of dementia in late adulthood. My father at the same age, however, is fortunate enough that his good health and indomitable spirit keeps him identifying with mature adulthood. He is a great role model for the activity theory of positive ageing: he has ambitious plans for the future, is on committees, exercises his body and mind through golf, swimming, exercise classes, and quiz evenings, and continually strives to develop and learn through golf lessons and playing competitive chess and bridge. No doubt he was influenced by his own father who learnt to swim in his 80s, evidencing the ability of the brain to generate new neurons and synapses after other neurons have degenerated (Snyder & Cameron, 2012). Perhaps even more remarkable has been my father's transition into carer in mature adulthood – not a natural role for him in their traditional 1950s marriage! In his 80s he learnt for the first time all my mother's conventional roles: cooking, cleaning, shopping, washing, ironing, and even arranging flowers! He has modelled Robert Atchley's (1989) "Continuity theory" of ageing that suggests that positive ageing involves maintaining a strong sense of self, personal history, and security and direction in life (helped by engaging with familiar skills, activities, and relationships), whilst continuing to evolve psychologically and socially despite changing and disturbing life events. Similar flourishing in mature adulthood (often through overcoming difficult circumstances) has been demonstrated by inspiring historical figures. The American folk artist, Grandma Moses, exhibited her work in Paris, Vienna, and at the MoMA in New York, despite only learning to paint at 78 after arthritis curtailed her embroidery; Nelson Mandela became President of South Africa aged 75 after 27 years of imprisonment for his fight against apartheid; Mother Teresa received the Nobel Peace Prize at 69; Peter Mark Roget was forced to retire from the Royal Society at 70 to make room for the younger generation, so instead published the enduring *Roget's Thesaurus* at 73 and oversaw each update until his death at 90; Charles Darwin published his revolutionary scientific masterworks from the ages of 50 to 73. Despite being ridiculed for researching the lowly earthworm, his work published six months before he died revolutionised horticulture, agriculture, and the global economy.

Challenges of mature adulthood

Such mature adults remain passionate, creative, and eager to learn. For many, however, the challenging adjustments involved in the transition into older age are hard to accept. There is still significant ageism in many individualist societies, acknowledged by the World Health Organization in 2016 when they created an "International Day of Older Persons" as part of a global campaign to challenge ageing stereotypes. Many older adults feel a reduced sense of usefulness and meaning in life as their longstanding work and relational roles shift and they feel overlooked in a youth-focused society. Difficulties can be experienced with physiological, mental, and sexual ageing and decline; ill-health or the ravages of dementia or cognitive impairment; a lack of structure and purpose in life through retirement or adjusting to the impact on their life of a partner retiring; redundancy; financial pressures; leaving the family home; an increasing number of bereavements including elderly parents, siblings, friends, or (particularly difficult) their life partner or children; a new identity as a grandparent or coming to terms with not being grandparents; facing the pain of estrangement from their adult children or supporting their children through difficulties with finances, relationships, work, child-rearing, divorce, or ill-health; caring for parents in late adulthood, whilst feeling the challenges of their own ageing, decline, and ever-nearing death. It is no wonder that Erikson (1968) described the work of this life stage as being about resolving the tension between integrity and despair. Some despair feels inevitable in this life stage – as in every other – but with enough support, overcoming the adversities of ageing can result in increased resilience, growth and integrity. As Ernest Hemingway (1929) writes, everyone is broken by the world, but afterwards, it is at the broken places that many are strongest.

Living well, laughing often, and loving much

At my parents' 90th birthday party, surrounded by their legacy of 24 children, grandchildren and great-grandchildren, my brother spoke of the things that had sustained them and our family through the struggles of life: optimism, passion, humour, and love. It reminded me of Bessie Anderson Stanley's (1904/1911) poem, "Success", which suggests that success is achieved by living well, laughing often, and loving much. Or as Eric Berne (1964) suggested, hopefulness, enthusiasm, or a lively interest in one's surroundings is the antidote to depression, and laughter the remedy for despair. Helping people who are struggling with the transition into mature adulthood often involves helping them find ways to overcome the adversities of ageing by learning to live life more fully, laugh and play more frequently, and love more deeply and maturely. This sentiment is echoed by Nietzsche (1883/1969), who argues that for maturity, humans have to go through the ordeal of the three metamorphoses of spirit: camel (capable of carrying the burdens of life), lion (freedom of autonomy, independent of duty), then child (innocence, vulnerability and a "sacred Yes" to enthusiasm in living life). He said that to do this, we must ten times a day overcome ourselves; reconcile ourselves with ourselves; discover truth; and laugh and be cheerful.

Optimism and hope

Hope and optimism are obviously harder with physical and mental challenges. Research shows that many adults gain modestly in agreeableness into their 70s (becoming more generous, acquiescent, and good-natured), and that retaining a flexible, optimistic approach to life in the face of adversity can contribute to psychological well-being, even with the more physical and cognitive challenges after 80 (Isaacowitz et al., 2016). Retaining a sense of pride in ageing and confronting internalised age discrimination can be helpful. We can learn much from cultures where older adults are treated with respect: the Inuit people of Canada describe elders as the head of the extended family and the "isumataq" or "one who knows things". A Japanese ritual called "kanreki" recognises the older person's seniority in the family and society, honouring its older citizens with an annual "Respect for the Aged Day". We must all take responsibility for confronting and fighting against implicit and explicit ageism in the same way we do for race, gender, or sexuality. And in so doing we can age with dignity, pride, and optimism. As suggested by the Welsh poet and writer, Dylan Thomas

(1937/2003) – who sadly died before mature adulthood – we should burn, rave and rage against old age and the dying of the light of life.

Finding new meaning

Burning, raving, and raging in mature adulthood is not about trying to cling on to youth but about finding new meaning and regeneration of the soul in later life. The mind and body may be experiencing some degeneration, but the soul can be regenerated in mature adulthood. Through accepting those aspects of ageing that cannot be changed, and raging, burning, and raving against those that can, the mature adult can enjoy "flourishing" rather than simply being "happy" (Seligman, 2011). In an interview by Aaron Hicklin in 1999, David Bowie suggests that:

> If you are pining for youth, I think it produces a stereotypical old man because you only live in memory, you live in a place that doesn't exist. Ageing is an extraordinary process where you become the person you always should have been.
>
> (Hicklin, 2016)

The awareness of limits of time can help mature adults place more emphasis on emotionally fulfilling relationships and on gratifying, meaningful experiences in the present. Once retired and if in good health, the mature adult may have more opportunity to pursue hobbies and creative activities, be involved in the lives of their grandchildren, or get involved in volunteering, mentoring, politics, gardening, continued learning, or the creative arts, all of which may provide a new sense of meaning and purpose in life. And of course, many in mature adulthood may continue to work with great satisfaction and accomplishment.

Passing wisdom on to others

This commitment to learning and rejuvenation is what transforms knowledge into wisdom. As Socrates was thought to have said, true wisdom comes to each of us when we realise how little we understand about life, ourselves, and the world around us. In *A Farewell to Arms*, Ernest Hemingway's (1929) poignant novel about love, war, and human resilience, he suggests that ageing well is about learning to understand the world and our place in it. First World War Lieutenant Frederic Henry is inspired by and learns from the wisdom of a 94-year-old former diplomat mentor, Count Greffi, who tells Frederic that the wisdom of old men is a fallacy if they prefer to grow careful rather than wise. It is an exaltation to those in mature adulthood to experiment, have courage, step out of their comfort zones, and to keep stretching themselves.

One of the ways we can do this is by offering a wealth of skills and life experience to society and younger generations. We can encourage mature adults who are struggling to find meaning in this life stage to give to others through mentoring, consultation, volunteering, becoming Justices of the Peace or community elders, offering something to aspire to, and offering comfort and continuity through holding the history that they have seen, survived, and learned from. Vaillant (2002) describes this as being society's Keepers of the Meaning, a vital lynchpin between past, present, and future. In doing so, both benefit from a mutual reciprocity. It is touching to see my son's relationship with his paternal grandparents, who, although now in their 80s, still have a youthfulness and playfulness about them that attracts him. At 22, and with a full work and social life, my son regularly makes time to speak with and visit them, enjoying the comfort, fun, and different perspectives on life that they offer as he explores his own beliefs and values as an emerging adult. Their years of dedication in playing with him, looking after him, challenging him, and supporting him through his parents' divorce, are culminating in a relationship that is mutually beneficial and precious to all of them; in a touching birthday card recently, they thanked him for bringing light into their life. As Fromm (1957) suggests:

> When one gives, he brings something to life in the other person, and this which is brought to life reflects back to him; in truly giving, he cannot help receiving that which is given back to him. Giving makes the other person a giver also, and they both share in the joy of what they have brought to life.
>
> (Fromm, 1957, pp. 20–21)

Existential guilt

Sometimes in a mature adult's search for meaning, they can suffer from a paralysing guilt and anxiety about how they have lived their life, a guilt that is an anxious sense of badness. Paul Tillich links anxiety with guilt, distinguishing between anxiety as a threat to objective existence (death), the threat to spiritual existence (meaninglessness), and the anxiety of self-condemnation (existential guilt).

> He is required to answer, if he is asked, *what he has made of himself*. He who asks him is his judge, namely he himself. The situation produces the anxiety which in relative terms is the anxiety of guilt, in absolute terms the anxiety of self-rejection or condemnation.
>
> (Tillich, 1952, p. 52)

We may need to help our clients come to terms with regrets, self-condemnation, and remorse. In doing so, it can be helpful to distinguish between three different types of guilt (Yalom, 1980). *Real guilt* emanates from an actual transgression that needs concrete or symbolic reparation: responsibility for a broken relationship or for regrets over work, lifestyle, or parenting. *Neurotic guilt* is a defensive, script-based guilt that is a disproportionate response to an imagined or minor transgression, or to something that actually belongs to someone else. It is often retroflected anger, aggression, or a wish for punishment, directing the emotions to self rather than outwards where they belong (in transactional analysis we might think of this as the rather outdated terminology of a "racket"). Through the intimacy and empathic challenge of the dialogic therapeutic relationship, we can help clients differentiate between real and neurotic guilt; identify how they may want to attempt to repair transgressions; confront possible contaminated beliefs; grieve adverse circumstances in childhood that have led to the self-alienation of neurotic guilt; and discover their authentic self.

Existential guilt, on the other hand, is a regret for not having fulfilled their potential: "The unused life, the unlived life in us" (Rank, 1945, as cited in Yalom, 1980, p. 278). Particularly common from mid-life onwards, it can be a positive constructive force, a useful reminder to us to take stock and make significant decisions about how we are going to use the rest of our life and fulfil our potential. What do we want our legacy to be? How do we want to be remembered? How can we best live well, laugh often, and love much? It is about taking responsibility for the present and the future in facing that one has not been authentic to self and thus has failed to fulfil authentic possibility: "Guilt is thus intimately related to possibility or potentiality" (Yalom, 1980, p. 277). In helping our clients distinguish between real, neurotic and existential guilt, we can help them find their "true" vocation and greater personal fulfilment. Kierkegaard (cited in May, 1977, p. 40) described this as the "will to be oneself", discovering the fundamental, permanent self underneath their adapted self or the "enduring I" (J.S. Mill, cited in Arendt, 1978, p. 9). In this way, the person can move from guilt and regret to acceptance and forgiveness, with hope for possibility in the future.

Michael

This was the journey for Michael, a handsome, well-groomed, and successful 66-year-old CEO of an international organisation. Michael had had an affair and was facing the consequences: his wife of 35 years and their children had disowned him, he faced losing his treasured home that he had spent his working life building, and he was facing the prospect of a lonely old age. I felt empathy for his brokenness, but also a distaste about his focus on his losses rather than any seeming empathy towards his wife, family, or the other woman whom he had discarded. I felt a disregard towards me when he took work calls in our sessions, and felt like a therapeutic prostitute when Michael, insisting on paying cash at the end of each session, stood over me and slowly counted out his money from a showy wad of bank notes. I began to wonder, somewhat cynically and a little guiltily, whether his wife had had a lucky escape. A book I enjoyed as a child and used to read to my own children flashed through my mind. *Mr Mean* (Roger Hargreaves, 1976) used to stay at home alone counting his money every night, until a firm but altruistic wizard appeared to teach him how to be kind. Was this what Michael needed from me? If so, I knew I was going to have to find more kindness towards him.

A love offering

This happened quite suddenly when Michael was unexpectedly and brutally made redundant. Experiencing his unadulterated vulnerability transformed our relationship and my feelings towards him. In utter desperation, he called me from a London bridge, considering throwing himself into the Thames. In that moment, the abyss of death seemed favourable to the isolation and destruction of his life as he had known it. His CEO persona was shattered, leaving a vulnerable, ageing man who was facing the despair and regrets of his life's decisions. I felt a flood of concern, love, and empathy and told him authentically that I cared that he lived and wished I was with him to hold his hand. He wept inconsolably as we metaphorically held hands and momentarily bridged the gap of his isolation. As Buber says, "A great relationship breaches the barriers of a lofty solitude, subdues its strict law, and throws a bridge from self-being-to-self-being across the abyss of dread of the universe" (Buber, 1965, p. 175). Perhaps being offered a bridge of relational connection helped Michael choose to live and leave his bridge of isolating despair. He came to see me the next day and at the end of the session reached for his wallet and said, "I owe you for yesterday". "No, that was my gift, Michael", I said tenderly and spontaneously, "A love offering". As I said it, I was taken back to my childhood biblical teachings about the "widow's mite", her humble impoverished offering of just two small copper coins being of far more value than the gold of the rich because it was given in love and generosity of spirit. It stopped Michael in his tracks. Money was a language of love to him, and his experience of life had been that you don't give or receive anything for free. He held out his hand wordlessly. I grasped it as I had longed to do when he was on the bridge, and we silently held each other's gaze in a fleeting moment that seemed to be outside of time, a reciprocal "small second of eternity" (Quinodoz, 2010, p. 8).

From fallen love to mature love

And so began Michael's long journey of facing his guilt and learning to live and love. Quinodoz believes that: "Growing old actively implies learning to love better" (Quinodoz, 2010, p. 193) and that it sometimes takes a whole life before we discover it. For many, mature adulthood is when we can finally learn to move from a symbiotic or "fallen" love to a mature love (Fromm, 1957) that is an attitude towards the world rather than just one individual. Rather than a symbiosis that is active (sadistic), or passive (masochistic) where neither party is whole or free, such mature love preserves one's integrity and individuality: "In love the paradox occurs that two beings become one and yet remain two" (Quinodoz, 2010, p. 17). Maslow (1962) describes this as the transition from an exploitative, self-serving love deriving from deficit, into a mature, un-needing love for the being of another person that is based on wanting to give rather than receive. It was mature love that I received when my cat died. It was mature love that I was able to offer Michael in his moment of need. It does not come from my own need, but in giving it freely, I inevitably also receive. As the priest advised Hemingway's Frederic: real love is when you want to do things for another person, you want to make sacrifices and serve them, and it is this that will make you happy. Mature love creates relational bridges that breaches the barriers of solitude.

The love of humour

At a celebration for their 50th wedding anniversary, my mother in mature adulthood passed on to the different generations of her family some of her wisdom about mature love. She said it was to listen to the unspoken communication and what was not being said, to look for the moments of love in action, and to find forgiveness when the other had fallen short. She gave the example of how, after an argument, she recognised that my father – not one to apologise – was sorry when she found him outside cleaning her car. Quick as a flash, he interrupted her speech with his characteristic lightning wit, heckling, "I wasn't sorry, I was just getting it ready to sell!". My Mum and the rest of the family roared with laughter. A defence against the intimacy of the small second of eternity? Perhaps. But also, an act of love, their shared humour uplifting, holding and sustaining their marriage and our family through the most joyous and darkest of times. A relational bridge. Their continued laughing together through my Mum's dementia has staved off despair and frustration, enabled the continued love in action of relentless caring, and provided connection with my Mum's core being. Laughing is a way of reconciling the ambiguities of love and hate, of tolerating the things we dislike in the other, of moving into a mature love that recognises that the people we love have not only qualities that delight us but also faults that distress us (Quinodoz, 2010). Humour in life and therapy helps us to love more fully, accepting a person's imperfections and moving to a love which accounts for the whole person and compensates both for the pain of existential isolation.

Mutual empathy

I explored with Michael what love meant for him and he gradually grieved the coldness of his parents' lack of love that was limited to their narcissistic pride in his achievements. Through my empathy, love, and challenge, he increasingly understood that love for him had been about power, status, lust, money, success, and domination. He had mistaken others' idolisation for love; in showing my humanity and his impact on me when he dismissed my feelings, I encouraged him to transcend his own self-concern and begin transforming "being loved" into "loving" (Fromm, 1952). My empathy for him was not enough for Michael: he also needed to be able to find empathy for me so that he could learn to love. The bridge needed to be built from both sides of the chasm. It was through the power of discovering each other through loving, mutual empathy – that was not always comfortable or easy – that Michael began to discover his true self and find new ways of being in relationship. This is described beautifully by Alfred Margulies:

> Telling one's narrative to another helps one find and constitute oneself: The narrator lives vicariously in the world of the listener as each tries to encounter the other's perspective... Empathy, in this respect, is a process which creates the self, either through the other or through empathy with oneself. That is, the self defines itself through empathy. In empathising with one another in the spiraling interchange, we name experience and invent a new language in metaphor to crystallize that which is not yet either in consciousness or existence. Here we create something together, make a link between disparate parts of experience and synthesize in new ways things already and almost there, but never before there in this way.
>
> (Margulies, 1989, pp. 142–143)

Guilt and responsibility

Michael's new narrative involved greater empathy for his family, which brought with it guilt and pain for his past exploitative actions. We differentiated between the neurotic guilt he felt that actually belonged to his parents, and the real guilt he felt for his adult choices. We also explored his anxiety that he was running out of time to put things right, and the regrets at the sacrifices he had made for the sake of his career. I encouraged him to view this existential guilt as a constructive guide to his future: how did he want to make the best use of his time left on earth? What did he value now as he approached 70? He wanted to make reparation for his previous decisions and decided to make use of his business experience by becoming a non-executive director of a charity that mentored unemployed young people. Most importantly, he desperately wanted to build bridges with his family and form a relationship with his grandchildren. We talked about how we can show love through small gestures, without expecting or demanding it in return. I encouraged him to notice the little ways that he experienced love every day: his mentee's smile of gratitude, the stranger running after him to return his dropped glove, his neighbour unexpectedly bringing him tomatoes from his greenhouse, the magical moment of eternity listening to an accomplished musician. In practicing noticing love, Michael was learning to integrate mature love into his life and being. As Quinodoz says: "We do need our whole life in order to learn, day after day, how to weave together frustrations and aggressiveness with tenderness and sensuality by means of everyday little things, in order to create love" (Quinodoz, 2010, p. 194).

Michael started demonstrating love to his children, sending them messages without expecting a reply, remembering important dates, writing to them to express his regrets, offering to look after his grandchildren and help them with their house maintenance. As they slowly started to accept his offered love and meet him part-way over the new bridge he was creating, Michael was tasting a different, more life-giving form of success. In her novel, To the Lighthouse, Virginia Woolf (1927) described these small daily miracles as matches that are struck unexpectedly in the dark that reveal the meaning of life. In mature adulthood, Michael was finding meaning through allowing light and love into his life, and appreciating more fully the small and unexpected moments of eternity that life and relationships could offer.

The red robin and the secret garden

As I approach the transition into mature adulthood I appreciate increasingly the small seconds of eternity, the little daily miracles, the matches struck unexpectedly in the dark. I think this capacity to savour the precious moments of life is a gift that older age offers. I relished this gift when my sister and I recently took my parents for a picnic to a peaceful, secluded garden. Our very own secret garden, where, in a little daily miracle, a cheeky little robin entertained us, made us laugh, and kept us company as we sat together. I noticed and appreciated with admiration in that garden how my father has grown in his capacity to love in his later years. Once a successful business executive providing financially for his family and being nurtured by my mother, I saw his newly developed patience, compassion, and tenderness as he now cares for her. And I saw my mother, now needing to be cared for by other people, still communicating her innate lifelong ability to love by trying to share her sandwiches with both us and the little robin. As we left that small second of eternity, I found myself singing an old song that my father used to play on the piano in my childhood: "When the red, red robin (Comes Bob, Bob, Bobbin' Along)" (written by Harry Woods, 1926). The lyrics urge us to wake up, get out of bed, listen to the sweet song of the red robin and cheer up, live, love, laugh, and be happy. As I approach mature adulthood, I remind myself to develop and savour those precious moments of birdsong, picnics in secret gardens, and of loving relationships. We never know whether we will reach the next life stage, but if I am fortunate enough to enter mature adulthood, I am keen to do so, like my role models, with an ever-growing capacity for living fully, laughing much, and loving maturely. I still have a lot to learn and a long way to go. I hope I continue to get the opportunity to practice.

Chapter 11

Late adulthood

Maintaining the indomitable core

My first experience of accompanying someone when they were dying was with my Grandad when I was a teenager. My parents were away and I was checking in on him as he hadn't been well with the lung condition, emphysema. When I rang, he was clearly finding it hard to breathe but being a proud Yorkshire man adamantly clinging on to his independence, he declined my offer to go round. I felt uneasy, and decided to go anyway. When he did not answer the door, I was terrified I would find him dead. He was still alive but in a very bad way. I called an ambulance and sat with him while we waited, watching him going increasingly grey. Everything within me wanted to get out of there. It was scary, horrific, anxiety-provoking, and I felt completely impotent as he struggled for each breath. But I knew it was right to stay with him; love overcame fear. When I finally left the hospital that night, we exchanged a look that I will never forget. Struggling to take the oxygen mask from his face and trying painfully to sit up, he said a simple and breathless, "Thank you". His eyes, however, said something so much more profound and meaningful than words could ever convey: love, gratitude, fear, pain. I hope my eyes communicated the same gratitude and love to him, for he died shortly after.

It is only now that I realise that in my naïve and inelegant way, I was accompanying my Grandad through his existential terror of death and dying. I hope that, despite the ignorance of my youth, being alongside him helped him feel less alone in his last days, and that, in some small way, I helped him to die more peacefully. For me, it was a spiritually and psychologically confronting life experience. Spinelli says:

> The extra-ordinary permits us a different view of the ordinary. This view may excite, arouse, fill with awe, horrify, terrify, take us away from our selves, put us closer in touch with our selves, make life worth living, or further destabilise our existential insecurities.
>
> (Spinelli, 2015, p. 100)

The experience brought me closer to death, dying, and existential fear, and showed me that I was capable of tolerating a lot more disturbance than I had

DOI: 10.4324/9781003475217-14

previously imagined. It probably unconsciously informed my growing interests in philosophy, theology, and psychology, and has certainly helped me as a psychotherapist and supervisor as I accompany those who are dying or in later life. It also normalised that, when we are faced with such demanding, soul-searching, and anxiety-provoking work, there will probably always be a sense of "wanting to get myself out of there" because it is infinitely more comfortable to look at life rather than death.

The challenges of decline in late adulthood

Too often when accompanying older people it is tempting to focus on the benefits of ageing as a defence against our own death anxiety, but this becomes increasingly difficult when working with the very old. The ravages of ageing in late adulthood mean that we cannot help but look in the mirror of our own decline when we accompany those in this life stage. Simone De Beauvoir offers a powerful confrontation: "We must stop cheating. The whole meaning of our life is in question in the future that is waiting for us... let us recognise ourselves in this old man or in that old woman" (De Beauvoir, 1977, p. 12). The future waiting for us in late adulthood, should we be fortunate enough to live that long, will most likely involve significant interrelated physical, mental, and psychological challenges: physical downturn can lead to deteriorating mental health, which can precipitate further giving up and physical shut-down in a vicious cycle of decline. This can be exacerbated if the older person is institutionalised and feeling isolated from the comfort of home, family, and friends. Physical illness, disability, bereavements, and increased frailty are common; changes in brain structure and the autonomic nervous system can lead to mental and cognitive decline which can affect memory, quality of sleep, immunity, and an increase in accidental falls; and a decline in sensory functions. Sight and hearing loss, in particular, can profoundly impact an older person's confidence, independence, and enjoyment of life as they can find it difficult to do the things they previously enjoyed, and can become increasingly isolated and dependent on others. In individualistic societies in particular, they may also be facing financial worries, fears about dementia or being placed in a nursing home, and age discrimination that involves stereotyping, objectification, being ignored, talked down to, or patronised (Nelson, 2011). Dr Kathryn Mannix, palliative care consultant and therapist, says that the elderly often accept their physical limitations as a price worth paying for living longer, but "Loneliness, many tell us, is a far harder burden than ill-health, and this is a sadness hidden in plain sight, a modern epidemic" (Mannix, 2022, p. 319). Depression is thus not uncommon in this life stage, yet paradoxically it is also probably the time in life where there is the greatest potent force towards self-awareness (Orbach, 1999; Yalom, 2011). The brain can compensate and adjust through reorganisation throughout life, and research has shown that when depressed old people are helped, they become more intellectually alert, have fewer accidents, need to be hospitalised less frequently, need less care, have a better social life, and somatic disorders ease (Berk, 2023). Therapy can therefore have significant benefits for very old clients, yet it is less common for them to get help. In England's National Health Service, a "miniscule" number of over 90s are in psychological treatment despite this being the fastest growing demographic group (Collins & Corna, 2018). I see this as a problem emanating potentially from both client and therapist.

Difficulties accessing therapy

Many very old people simply do not think of or seek therapy. Therapy was not a common phenomenon when current older generations were young, they may believe it is only for those with major disorders, and there are often lingering stigmas around needing help, sharing feelings, or being a burden. Internalised age discrimination may leave them feeling that they are not worth the investment in therapy, that their difficulties are simply age-related, or that limited time left means that change is not possible. They may also find it hard to access therapy because of transport, disability, financial difficulties, or struggles with technology, particularly if they are in hospital or a care home. They may fear opening up a "can of worms", anxious about facing death or missed opportunities. In addition, having a younger therapist that may be the same age as their children or grandchildren can evoke painful reminders of their younger years, envy of the therapist's generativity, or anxiety that they will not have the life experience or spiritual awareness necessary to understand them.

The challenges for the therapist

The reality is that many therapists are also anxious about their competency of working with people in this life stage. They may be cautious or feel inadequate because of the age difference and their lack of life experience and may feel unable to tolerate the transferential dynamics that evoke for the therapist difficult childhood memories, issues to do with parenting their own children, the loss of deceased parents, or fear of their own parents' ageing or dying. They may voice concerns about the ethics of potentially opening up old wounds for the client with limited years ahead of them, which might cover unconscious biases, beliefs, and fears about older people and a conscious or non-conscious belief that working with older people is a poor investment of time (Kastenbaum, 1964). Perhaps because of their own spiritual paucity, the therapist may not see or understand the potential spiritual benefits of ageing, where meaning can be discovered by devotion to the sacred (McFadden, 1999) and a transcendent perspective on self, life and death. Often it comes down to a fear of difference – the "everyday mysticism" of old age (Atchley, 1997) – and an ignorance or avoidance of similarities, death and ageing.

Uncovering prejudices

Unconscious prejudice might blind us to the possibility that some things we and society put down to old age – accidents, somatic illnesses, mental decline – could actually be an unconscious cry for help and an unspoken communication of unsupported mourning, grieving, depression, and death anxiety. We need to keep reflecting about our own unconscious drives: perhaps we might also objectify older people by non-consciously attempting to use them to repair our own past relationships or to provide care for parental figures that we had failed to do in our own lives. We need to be careful to account for the context of age but not define anyone by their life stage. We must remind ourselves that every person and every moment of every life is precious, irreplaceable, and unique, whilst remembering the particular significance of time for those in very old age: The focus is "finding out how each different individual is able to understand the many experiences they have had in their lives and how they are preparing themselves to harvest that learning in preparation for the final summary of the ending" (van Deurzen & Adams, 2016, p. 193).

Impactful therapy in very old age

If therapist and older client have the opportunity, desire, and courage, the work has the potential to be deeply impactful for both. Kathryn Mannix gives a poignant account of the mutuality of working with a 98-year-old dying woman, who "regrets that she has lived past being useful and mobile". As a doctor on her rounds, she had an uncomfortable menopausal flushing at the woman's bedside. Despite being desperately frail, the older woman offered her doctor a fan and some maternal advice about the menopause. Kathryn noted the older woman's capacity, even at her life's end, for offering wisdom, kindness, and mentoring, and in Kathryn being willing to receive her gift, the woman became momentarily whole again. She movingly reflected:

> I feel an awareness of our similarities, rather than of the differences imposed by age and ill-health. Our elderly are so easily dispossessed, stripped of their personhood by eyes like mine too young to value their accumulated wisdom, experience and patience. I have learned an important lesson from this very frail and aged woman.
>
> (Mannix, 2022, p. 319)

Young and old need to be open to learning from and giving to each other. I was once on a tutor team with a talented and experienced teacher in her 70s. I was keen to learn from her but felt her distance so retreated myself. It was when she courageously acknowledged her envy of me for being on the ascendency in my career whilst she was approaching retirement that we could move into a mutuality of relating where I could benefit from her experience and wisdom and she could gain meaning from mentoring me.

With mutuality, the breadth and depth of therapeutic possibility also extends rather than diminishes in older adulthood. With the offering of our self in authentic relationship, impactful therapy with the very old can involve offering companionship, easing aloneness, sharing the joys and despairs of humanity; raising awareness, helping them search for and discover a better relationship with self and other, providing a witness to their life's narrative; enabling the integration of memories and the delight of discovering more of their internal world; coming to terms with the shadow side of life, assistance with mourning, support with accepting the unsolvable and unreconcilable, holding helplessness; helping them live more fully in their time remaining, savouring every precious moment of life, experiencing joy and laughter, learning to love; deepening spiritual awareness, silently accompanying, finding meaning; facing regrets, journeying to a place of peace and forgiveness, help with dying, and preparing for the "end goal" of death (Jung, 1931/1970). We may never know how, but we will always find meaning and growth from being alongside another in this profound and spiritual journey. As Robert Browning (1864/2023, p. 207) invites enticingly in his poem, "Rabbi Ben Ezra", "Grow old along with me! The best is yet to be, the last of life, for which the first was made."

Finding wisdom in life's shadow

The "best" of the last stage of life has often been seen as the achievement of integrity and wisdom. Vaillant (2002) suggested that this included the ability to reflect on one's life with satisfaction, peace and gratitude, whilst Erikson (1968) proposed that it was about resolving the conflict between integrity and despair. Erikson and his wife, Joan (Erikson & Erikson, 1997), said that overcoming different psychosocial tensions at different life stages would lead to the development over a lifetime of character strengths such as hope, will, purpose, competence, fidelity, love, and care, with wisdom and integrity the ultimate goal and prize of old age. After Erik had died, however, Joan realised they had been naïve in their eight stages, and described how others might see wisdom and integrity in an old person that they do not feel in themselves because disintegration of mental and physical health can lead to despair and isolation. She therefore added a ninth life stage – Very Old Age – and proposed that the goal of this life stage was to come to terms with the shadow side (dystonic) of the conflicts of the previous eight stages with which life confronts us all, particularly in old age: mistrust, shame, role confusion, isolation, stagnation, despair, guilt, and inferiority.

It is important, however, that we remember that conflict and tension are sources of growth, strength, and commitment and that we do not pre-empt the older person's experiences of gains and losses. Some may be preoccupied with their struggle with decline, others may consider that the wisdom gained outweighs the losses of old age (van Deurzen & Adams, 2016). Perhaps wisdom in this life stage comes to those who have in life suffered, overcome, and learned to accept that loss and unwanted change is an inevitable – but manageable – part of human existence. With this wisdom, the very real challenges of old age (if fortunate enough to arrive there) might be a little more tolerable.

Facing death, dying, and ageing

The realities of impending death, however, can be daunting (to say the least) for even the wisest people, and can come with a sense of disbelief. As the elderly composer played by Michael Caine in Paolo Sorrentino's film, "Youth" exclaimed: "I've become old and I don't know how I got here". Helping people make sense of "how they got here" and reassessing their life's achievements, disappointments, joys, regrets, and losses will be part of therapy with the older adult. Paradoxically, the "old" are often more able to address ageing and dying than the young, and with those approaching death, it is no longer a theoretical discussion but a very personal acknowledgement of *my* death (Cooper & Adams, 2005). They may be asking themselves: "Is it okay to have been me?", and coming to terms with regrets can be particularly disturbing and confronting work. Younger therapists might fear older clients holding up a mirror to their own future and fears of ageing, mortality, or dying. Avoiding the topic or simply focusing on positive elements of getting old, however, will compound the client's isolation, and we need to examine carefully and with humility our own avoidance because of potential death anxiety and fear of ageing. If they are open to it, the young can learn a great deal about ageing from the old. They can help those younger than them to confront their own anxieties and fears about the transient nature of life, ageing and mortality, and help them make the most of the remaining time they have in life.

Maintaining the "indomitable core" of self

Whilst it is crucial to face death, we must not be overwhelmed by it, and need to remember that not every issue older people bring to therapy is connected directly to death and dying. It is important that there is a focus on living life as fully as possible in the context of there being limited time remaining. Ricoeur (2007) describes this as seeing the "still-alive" person and reminding those that are coming to the end of their life that they still have resources that sustain them. It is important that older people are enabled to preserve their autonomy whenever possible. Joan Erikson (Erikson & Erikson, 1997) expresses this as maintaining their self's "indomitable core". I once made the mistake of suggesting a vigorous activity was not age-appropriate to my 87-year-old father. "Don't make me old before my time!" he chided me. I considered myself told! And what a great role model for old age, to fiercely defend that truly indomitable core.

Out of care, concern, rescuing, or discrimination, family members and caregivers often promote excessive dependency in old age, which can unnecessarily and prematurely take away their autonomy. Alternatively, the older person may need more support but can be so scared of losing control and independence that they do not accept or ask for help when they need it. We can help them explore the support they want and need, offer direction to services and charities that may be helpful, and challenge them to decide how they want to adapt to fit their changing capabilities and maximise joy and sense of purpose by prioritising their most treasured activities. We need to encourage those in late adulthood to find and nurture their innate resources to that they can tap into their life force, not just focus on who they no longer are or what they can no longer do. Even my mother, in the later stages of dementia and with an increasingly childlike dependency, still has a resourcefulness that displays her lifelong indomitable core. She finds ways to connect through a surprisingly still-quick wit and continued avid interest in others. Although she does not retain my answers or even remember who I am, our souls connect and communicate love and, in that way, I act as a witness to her own resourcefulness and life force. Relatedness helps her discover, express, and know herself once more. Quinodoz describes it beautifully as looking carefully to see the resources that are still present and being able to see the person as a "pure presence" like a tree: a presence that we "could feel, without knowing how to describe it" (Quinodoz, 2010, p. 86).

Forming a narrative of their lives

Being a witness to their resourcefulness helps older people open up their internal world, describe their lives in whatever way they are able to, and thus know themselves better. They can also internalise the therapeutic relationship and appreciate more fully life's other internalised positive relationships, which can help allay painful solitude: "The presence of good internal objects acts as a counterbalance to the loss of external objects. We can withstand loneliness better if our internal world is inhabited" (Quinodoz, 2010, p. 88). The integration and remembrance of positive relationships and experiences enables us to feel more fully connected to the environment, wider world, and the transpersonal. This is important for coming to terms with death, which involves letting go of our unique individuality in a finite world and embracing our return to being part of the boundaryless mystery of eternity. Vaillant describes this as coming to terms with the fact that we all one day cease to be a special and "terminally unique" wave, but that "ageing allows us to feel part of the ocean" (Vaillant, 2002, p. 278). Helping older people form a narrative of their lives assists them in finding coherence and completeness between past, present and future as they contemplate moving from wave to ocean:

> Each period in our life, with its dramatic moments and its joys, is important; we need to find all of them vibrating within us in our present time in order to perceive the originality of our existence. Besides, we see that in some

elderly people their childhood, adolescence and adulthood are all contained in the age they have at present; bringing all of these phases together gives a certain harmony to their old age.

(Quinodoz, 2010, p. 29)

Reminiscing and a sense of nostalgia as they reintegrate lost memories becomes particularly important for the older person in their story-telling. We need patience, respect, a genuine interest, and healthy curiosity about the context in which they have lived and worked and hold the minutiae and details of their life story with an "attitude of meaning" (Mowzat, 2005, p. 11). Reminiscing helps the very old person make meaning and better reconcile change and continuity; they can recognise their gradual evolution as a person through the changes of their lives and the world, but that they have also essentially stayed the same person from birth to death. As they slowly piece together a more coherent narrative they can more fully appreciate how the past has shaped who they are and who they will become in whatever time they have left. We must remember that there is always hope for the ongoing creation of something new out of something old, right up until death: "We can constantly go on creating our life in the present moment like a work of art... From time to time, each of us can see that 'one must have chaos in one to give birth to a dancing star'" (Nietzsche, 1883/1969, Part 1, v.5).

Developing spiritual awareness

Seeing our life as a work of art or our self as a dancing star is particularly challenging if in the depths of the profound loneliness, despair, and isolation that can accompany ageing. Having lost previous ways of obtaining connection, meaning and purpose because of the decline of old age, Mannix suggests we must ask, "...How do we enable them to experience satisfaction and self-worth, not in return for making a contribution but simply for being their unique selves?" (Mannix, 2022, p. 319). I believe the answer is in mutuality and in enabling the older person to be able to make a difference to *me*. I must be open to offering my humanity, my heart, and my soul to the relationship in order that I can be moved, touched, and confronted. As they approach life's final boundary of death, I find that therapeutic boundaries become more diffuse, and offering my presence and showing kindness, generosity, and sensitivity are more important to me than rigidity. Some boundary issues may arise because of memory lapses, hospital visits, transport issues, or illnesses, but time in general also becomes less about clock-watching and more about the concept of past, present, and future in the context of eternity. Particularly if I visit my older clients at home, in hospital or care home, the presence of the boundary of death can make our sessions start feeling more like pastoral care, companionship, or spiritual guidance.

I make no apology for enjoying these shifting boundaries and the deepening spiritual connection of our relationship at these times. It can feel as though we are transcending time, life, and death as we slow down and find in the "small moments of eternity" together the little things that might be more usually missed in the busyness of life or the rigid 50-minute therapy session: moments of love and tenderness; an appreciation of each other's presence as we listen to the silence; holding hands; short strolls into the garden; gently or playfully singing a song together. Joan Erikson (Erikson & Erikson, 1997) suggests we can heighten spiritual awareness – perhaps the greatest potential resource for those in later adulthood – through touch, play, activity, joy, song, and humility. She describes this as "gerotranscendence" (Tornstam, 2005), a psychospiritual developmental theory of positive ageing. Tornstam, a Swedish sociologist, said that those in very old age can be helped by a focus on what is above and beyond and a redefinition of the self in relationship to others and the universe. They can discover meaning in this stage of life by maintaining devotion to the sacred, which can often involve a spirituality that moves from an outward to an inward focus. Vaillant (2002) says this can come from the simplicity of life and the capacity to be internally quiet. This is echoed by other religious, spiritual, and analytic writings: the Hindu concept of life stages suggests that when we become grandparents we should turn away from the world and take up spiritual interests (Radhakrishnan, 1989). Christian teachings also urge spiritual renewal as death approaches: "Those who wait on the Lord shall renew their strength; They shall mount up with wings like eagles..." (Isaiah 40:31, New King James Version, 1982), whilst Jung (1963) said that old age was not a waiting room looking backwards, but a time for making ourselves ready for whatever comes next after death.

Choosing forgiveness and reconciliation

Making ourselves ready for death will inevitably stir old regrets and grievances, unresolved relational disruptions and other unfinished business, as well as unexpressed gratitude and appreciation. In the psychological and existential literature this is often framed as a striving or need for "self-acceptance", "self-love", "closure", "letting-go" or "reconciliation" (Ransley & Spy, 2004). What is sometimes missing is the concept of forgiveness for self and other, a pre-requisite for all of these other concepts. Beneath any challenges with relational connection or unfinished business is often a difficulty with the capacity to forgive. Authentic forgiveness offered in purity of spirit is at the heart of human existence, and enables a level of healing, peace, inner stillness, restoration of relationship, healthy endings, and creative new beginnings. At no time is this more important than at the end of our lives when we may feel a strong urge to tie up loose ends as we face our final ending of death.

And yet psychotherapists are sometimes reluctant to engage with forgiveness because of negative religious, cultural, or political connotations. They may fear colluding with minimising the reality of the offence or of the difficult feelings associated with it. They may see some efforts of forgiveness as a defensive way of holding on to victimhood and self-flagellation, or as a destructive striving to return to a harmful relationship or even for passive-aggressive revenge. All of these can be true, and I am certainly not saying that forgiveness involves staying in an abusive or coercive relationship. But remaining stuck in unforgiveness can also be harmful, and research has shown significant neurophysiological and psychological benefits to authentic forgiveness: decreases in heart rate and respiratory rate, less anxiety and depression, reduced negative thoughts, behaviours, and feelings of anger and hostility, improved self-esteem, improved sleep patterns, decreased levels of stress hormones, and a greater sense of empowerment (Gubi, 2015). In short, genuine forgiveness reduces our own suffering and increases our wellbeing, and the end of someone's life can be infinitely more peaceful and freeing if we can help people explore whether there is anyone – including themselves – that they would like to forgive.

What is forgiveness?

It is helpful to consider what we mean by forgiveness, as there are many misconceptions. Enright and Coyle state that forgiveness should be differentiated from pardoning, condoning, excusing, forgetting, and denying. It is "a willingness to abandon one's right to resentment, negative judgment and indifferent behaviour toward one who unjustly hurt us, whilst fostering the undeserved qualities of compassion, generosity, and even love toward him or her" (Enright & Coyle, 1998, pp. 46–47). It is a gradual letting go of bitterness, overwhelming anger, or the search for revenge. Forgiving does not mean that we will stay in a relationship with someone, that we will not feel a myriad of difficult feelings, or that we will not seek appropriate justice. It is right that perpetrators of abuse experience consequences of their actions. But we can still achieve intrapsychic reconciliation through forgiveness, even if interpersonal reconciliation is not possible or desirable. Sometimes we may need to work through the hate, pain, and guilt of past psychic wounds and the forgiveness for our early caregivers before we can forgive those in the present or more recent past (Anderson, 2014).

Many people who say they cannot forgive are often not yet in a position to imagine that the hurt or bitterness will ever subside, and with the most serious of offences it may take years for these feelings to shift enough for someone to even consider forgiveness. Forgiveness takes time – sometimes a lifetime – and is an ongoing process, particularly when we continually experience the consequences of the offender's actions. Disturbing feelings about the offence will inevitably re-emerge, even when we have chosen to forgive, but it is not a polarity of resentment *or* forgiveness; both can co-exist. Feelings will usually gradually lessen in intensity and we can become less consumed by them, re-deciding to continue on the forgiveness path.

It is easier to choose to forgive when we can recognise some common humanity with the person who offended us, when we can acknowledge the good and bad in us all, and that we all have times when we do not deserve forgiveness. We need empathy and inclusion to reach authentic forgiveness: the capacity to be grounded in one's own experience and at the same time to enter the world of the other. This empathy is reliant on us apportioning appropriate responsibility for choices, behaviours, and regrets, and letting go of inappropriate guilt and judgement. Forgiving others and forgiving self are intertwined:

> Forgiveness occurs when truth has broadened… There is the capacity to bear complexity and ambivalence, where I am both good and bad; you have offended and hurt me but you have your good parts too, or your badness can be understood, and above all we are both part of the human race.
>
> (Anderson, 2014, p. 75)

The ability to forgive is learned, develops, and changes through the life stages and over the course of personality development, with older people tending to be more forgiving as they age (Ermer et al., 2022). But forgiveness is also not an "either/or" paradigm, and everyone has the choice to not forgive or to refuse forgiveness. We need to be sensitive to personal, historical, religious, and cultural context, and not to try to influence an elderly person to forgive, but to empower them in considering their options and thinking through how forgiving or withholding forgiveness will impact them in their final stage of life.

Louisa

Louisa, a frail 86-year-old widow, came to see my supervisee, Bea (a psychotherapist in her mid-30s), because of feelings of isolation, difficulties in relationships, and low mood. She had broken relationships with her two daughters, and reported consistently being "let down" and avoided by people in the church she attended. Bea could understand why: she found Louisa difficult to connect with and described her as at times "prickly", "fractious", "controlling" and "unforgiving". Bea found it hard to get it right for Louisa. She said she felt like Louisa was Goldilocks in the house of the three bears: everything and everybody was too hard, too soft, too hot, too cold, too big, too small. Yet unlike Goldilocks, Louisa rarely found anything "just right", and had little empathy or forgiveness for those she considered had wronged her. Bea discovered that Louisa had grown up with unbearable loneliness, being adopted by a couple who found her an inconvenience and showing her little love or affection. These dynamics seemed to be repeating in the present but Louisa had little interest in making links with the past or grieving historical abandonments. "I don't think I can help her," Bea lamented in supervision, "It's too late for her to change". I challenged Bea: "Maybe it's not so much about change but more about acceptance of the life she has lived". Bea was incredulous. "How can she accept her life?" she responded, "there's nothing for her to live for". "So maybe it's about Louisa coming to terms with that?", I suggested, "Maybe she needs your help to find a way to accept that life is challenging and has been full of disappointments, and make peace with that before she dies".

Intrusion and fear

Bea and I played with the analogy of the Goldilocks fairy-tale and the parallels with Louisa. How Goldilocks had been searching for home and had intruded without invitation into the lives of others: broken into the bears' home, eaten their food, broken their chair, and slept in their bed, all in the quest for perfection. Yet when the bears returned, there was no possibility of forgiveness, belonging, and acceptance because she fearfully ran away. Might Bea's offer of love be Louisa's last opportunity for repair, reconciliation, and to fulfil unmet desires? Or would she again run away in fear? "Perhaps your challenge to Louisa is to offer your love and humanity; I don't think it's ever too late to have a different experience,", I offered, "but whether she chooses to receive it in the time she has left is up to her".

Offering humanity

Louisa's opportunity to receive Bea's love came shortly afterwards in an unwanted and unexpected way. Louisa was unusually late to her session. When Bea answered the door, she was met by a flustered stranger who said that Louisa was asking for her. She had fallen over in the street, and when Bea arrived, Louisa was in shock and clearly injured. Bea covered her with blankets and Louisa seemed noticeably reassured by her presence, holding her hand while they waited for the ambulance. When the paramedics arrived, Louisa grabbed Bea's hand more firmly and looked her desperately in the eye: "please will you come with me?", she implored. Bea was faced with an anxious ethical dilemma, paralleling the unresolved tensions of Louisa's 86 years of life: Aloneness versus relationship; safety versus risk; autonomy versus dependence.

"I was so torn, Rachel," Bea told me afterwards. "I couldn't leave her alone when she needed me and was finally asking for relationship, but I kept thinking of ethics boards. I didn't know what to do, I didn't have any experience to draw on". Tears welled in my eyes as Bea told me cautiously that she had chosen to go with her to hospital and had stayed for hours until Louisa's neighbour arrived. "You did have experience", I responded gently, "you had your humanity".

Reparation

Bea's gift to Louisa of her love, care, and relational risk was a profound and creative spiritual experience that transcended her role as a therapist and touched all three of our souls. She continued to visit Louisa in hospital and, when she was discharged but still too frail to come to her therapy room, was moved and surprised when Louisa also took a relational risk and invited Bea into her home. Bea and I couldn't help smiling at the mutuality and creativity of the sharing of each other's homes, and the significance that rather than intruding uninvited into the bears' home, "Goldilocks" was inviting the "Bear" into hers! Being careful not to intrude herself, but wanting to help Louisa tell her story and continue creating her "life's work of art", she sensitively asked about the books on the shelves and the family photos that adorned Louisa's walls. Louisa gradually opened up about her life history, her regrets and disappointments, bitterness and grief, and her previously unexpressed love of poetry. She could no longer read the small print of many of her books, but she asked Bea to read her favourite poems out loud. Sharing her old loves with this young woman who was poignantly of a similar age to her estranged daughters, Louisa finally found a small taste of a love that was "just right" amidst the devastation of lost love and opportunity. And in sharing her home, memories and poetry with her, perhaps she was able to start learning to love and to find a way to begin making her own internal reparation for the broken family relationships.

Peace

Louisa never reconciled with her daughters and did not openly acknowledge forgiveness of herself or them, but Bea felt a growing aura of peace in their time together. As Louisa grew increasingly frail, they experienced longer and longer periods of reflective silence where they seemed to simply enjoy each other's presence. Louisa's last gift to Bea before she died was a poem called "The Fountain: A Conversation" by William Wordsworth (written in 1799). This time Louisa was determined that she would read it herself:

> We talked with open heart, and tongue Affectionate and true,
> A pair of friends, though I was young, And Matthew seventy-two....
> ...`Thus fares it still in our decay: And yet the wiser mind
> Mourns less for what Age takes away, Than what it leaves behind.
>   (Wordsworth, 1994, p. 581)

Through the faltering and emotional recitation of the poet's reflections on relationship, life, death, and grief, it seemed that Louisa was acknowledging her own losses, whilst telling Bea that she appreciated her companionship in her last months of life and that, in her own special way, she loved her.

Section 3

Death and life

Chapter 12

Death and endings

Balancing life and death

Death, continuity, and change

Death is painful. I am currently experiencing the rawness of grief following the recent death of a dear friend; a grief so multi-faceted that I am sometimes confused about where my pain emanates from. I feel an acute stabbing loss for the solid and reliable presence of the man with whom I had a 25-year friendship, his absence making me face my existential aloneness with more crystal clarity. Undoubtedly, this also taps into archaic grief (conscious and unconscious), reopening wounds of abandonment, loss, and aloneness that usually lie dormant. I mourn for his life cut short, for the harsh reality that he will not see his grandchild, born a few weeks before he died, grow up. It is a painful reminder that our lives can end at any moment and that when we are dead, we will never know the next chapter of the life stories of those we love. I grieve for his wife and children, the sometimes-haunted look of anguish etched on their faces a reminder of the inevitability of pain and suffering in life, and the almost impossible task we have in coming to terms with the constancy and inevitability of unwanted change. I grieve for the world, for the loss of his immense skill, wisdom, and life experience, knowing that, with his absence, the world is a poorer place. I am reminded of our lack of control over death, and feel an existential anxiety and despair about the threats to human existence through wars, conflicts, climate change, competition, greed, power, and the destructive forces of humanity. My anguished soul reminds me that grief is an inevitable aspect of existence, located simultaneously in the past, present, and future.

The day after my friend's funeral, I visited a local garden, a favourite haunt of both our families since the birth of our children. As I walked and cried, I was flooded with memories from my adult life to which this garden had been witness. The joy of my firstborn learning to crawl across the grass, summer picnics under the trees, snowdrop walks promising the hope of spring, Christmas carol concerts and mulled wine, my children finding conkers and playing hide-and-seek with their grandparents, winter light festivals with their partners when they emerged into adulthood. Also, the pain of returning without my husband after our separation, or with my Mum after a dementia

DOI: 10.4324/9781003475217-16

diagnosis, or my young niece whilst undergoing cancer treatment, and now after the death of my friend, the garden beholding the next chapter of my life story. The garden offers a reassuring sense of continuity, familiarity, comfort, and a holding presence through these turbulent times of joy and pain. Yet every time I go, something has changed: a Japanese garden created in old wasteland, an old familiar climbing tree blown over in the gales, the constant growth and decay of the ever-changing seasons. And every time I go, *I* have also changed, I am not the same person as the last time I went. The Greek philosopher Heraclitus (n.d., cited in Graham, 2023) famously said: "No man ever steps in the same river twice, for it's not the same river and he's not the same man". Growth and decay poignantly remind us that we cannot control change, and that we are constantly faced with the existential tension between change and continuity: the greatest paradox of change is that it is the *only* constant in our lives. We *will* experience change continually: sometimes expectedly, willingly, consciously, sometimes unexpectedly, unwillingly, unconsciously. Ernesto Spinelli (2015) describes three experiences of change:

1 *Spontaneously accepted changes* that are barely in our awareness and can be integrated effortlessly into our lives and sense of self without defence (the subtle change in our bodily cells or our relational being every time we encounter another).
2 *Reflectively accepted changes* that enthuse, excite, shake, move, and/or surprise us, whether positively or negatively. We can reflect on them and ultimately accept their impact upon our relational being (becoming ill, falling in love, failing an exam, becoming a parent, ending with a client).
3 *Reflectively troubling or rejected changes* that we consider unwanted, unfair, disturbing, unacceptable, and/or intolerable, or involve our perceived incapacity to bring about desired change. These experiences, and our attempts to reject, prevent, reduce, or deny them, are often what bring people to therapy or consultation, and cause the most disruption, division, and impasse in relationships, families, work places, educational establishments, and our communities (death, divorce, ageing, relational breakdown, redundancy, war, conflicts, oppression).

Change as movement-towards-death

Whether we see potential changes as reflectively accepted, reflectively troubling, or outright rejected will be different for all of us, depending on our genetic make-up; our personal histories and relationships; our unique personalities, beliefs and values; and our relationship with change and power. What is common to all of us, however, is that change is disruptive and reminds us consciously or non-consciously of our "movement-towards-death" (Heidegger, 1927/2010). With every change there is an existential death of the being-who-was (Spinelli, 2015) and we need to let go of our old self so that the new self can emerge. The uncertainty of who the new self will be and how we will be impacted by the change, as well as the reminder of the final letting go of self in death, creates anxiety:

> It can be recognized that our reflective experience of ongoing change, and our responses to it, is intimately tied to death anxiety in that any instance of change requires the "death" of whatever – or whoever – had existed prior to having undergone that change.
>
> (Spinelli, 2015, p. 51)

This is so painful for some people that they find ways to defend against their death anxiety. Our role is to help our clients, supervisees, and trainees come to terms with change, their existential anxiety, and their own death, so that they can live more authentic, vital, and fulfilling lives.

Death and transactional analysis

Death anxiety, however, has been somewhat avoided in transactional analysis (TA), and Berne skirted over endings in his writing. Perhaps this is because of Berne's own history with the premature death of his father when Berne was just ten years old, the subsequent loss of his home, and the emotional and physical withdrawal of his mother through depression. Berne (1966) described three different types of therapeutic endings (accidental, resistant, and therapeutic) – to which Tudor (1995) added "enforced" endings – but his treatment plan did not outline how or why to work with endings. His focus on change was that of script cure, neglecting the existential anxiety of change as movement-to-wards-death. Heathcote describes, "a gaping hole regarding loss, grief, mourning, and melancholia in the transactional analysis theory developed by Berne" (Heathcote, 2016, p. 240). Mothersole (1996) agrees, proposing that Berne's focus on positive change, autonomy, and script cure at the expense of endings in life and psychotherapy was a consequence of TA's development during the prosperity of 1960s West Coast America.

Berne did not avoid writing about death completely, however. In *What Do You Say After You Say Hello?* (Berne, 1972/1992), he talked about the human destructive forces of death ("mortido") that are universally present alongside the life force of "eros" (I return to both in the next chapter). He described death as a "transaction", our imagined "deathbed scene" being part of our life script (Berne, 1972/1992) and hinted at the inevitability of death and the somewhat meaninglessness of life in his deterministic view of script, games, and time-structuring: "Human life is mainly a process of filling in time until the arrival of death, or Santa Claus, with very little choice, if any, of what kind of business one is going to transact during the long wait" (Berne, 1964, p. 162). He seemed to become increasingly philosophical as his own death approached, musing about whether he was a piano player whose playing (life) was being determined by a piano roll (script) or whether he was "a brave improviser facing the world alone" (Berne, 1972/1992, pp. 276–277). Yet he did not acknowledge any existential death anxiety: "I wait with interest and anticipation – and without apprehension – for the next notes to unroll their melody, and for the harmony and discord after that. Where will I go next?" (Berne, 1972/1992, pp. 276–277). Tragically, by the time this was published, Berne was already dead.

Other TA authors have since filled something of the gaps left by Berne and have written about bereavement, loss, grief, mourning, endings, and transitions (Cornell, 2013, 2014; Erskine, 2014; Garcia, 2012; Heath, 2014; Lankford, 1980; McQuaid, 2021; Stewart, 1996; Tudor, 1995; Welford, 2014). The denial of death was touched upon by Goulding & Goulding (1979) in writing about "Goodbyes", but their focus is on fully acknowledging the death of others through a redecision process rather than facing the inevitability of our own death. The TA literature that specifically addresses death anxiety is sparse: Conway (1978) describe counterscript messages and driver behaviour as coping mechanisms that enable us to deny our most primitive fears around our non-being; Bowater (2008) gives an account of helping a man in his 90s face his impending death and associated terror; and, based on the philosophical Vedantic worldview from India, Suriyaprakash and Geetha (2014) suggest that spiritual integration is an antithesis to fear of death. It is clear that TA could benefit from leaning further into an existential approach to death and the inevitable anxiety that surrounds it, so that we can help ourselves and our clients face change, death, and endings with greater courage and equanimity.

What is death anxiety?

Death anxiety is the anxiety experienced in daily life caused by the uncertainty, anticipation, and fear of death. It can be about the ending of one's own life but also others' lives, the end of relationships, the world's existence, or of the ending of strongly held values, beliefs, hopes, or aspirations. It can also involve anxieties about the possible pain and suffering of dying, ageing, or circumstances that confront one with the idea of death, such as an accident or ill-health. We can also feel anxiety about leaving others behind when we die, being concerned for their well-being, their grief, or our inability to be able to continue to care for them. We can fear missing out on aspects of life that have not yet been lived, or goals we have not yet managed to fulfil. As Sartre laments:

> Death is an outrage that comes to me from outside and wipes out my projects. Death cannot be prepared for, or made my own; it's not something to be resolute about, nor something to be incorporated or tamed. It is not one of my possibilities but "the possibility that there are for me no longer any possibilities".
>
> (Sartre, 1946/1953, p. 687)

The growing awareness of our mortality and that we will never be able to do all the things we want to with our life can lead to great existential angst around the other givens of human existence. We can feel the burden of the freedom and responsibility to make the right choices with our finite time, as well as a desperate search to make meaning of the life we have left. Spinelli (2015) argues that death anxiety is an all-encompassing presence throughout our experience of living and is grounded in relatedness; the fear of the ultimate separation of death can therefore induce an overwhelming sense of aloneness and isolation.

Death challenges the fantasy that we have control over our lives. We grapple with the tension between certainty of death and uncertainty of when or how we will die and whether there is any afterlife, and we often struggle to accept that we have no control that one day our "being" will end. This thought is an outrage! British philosopher and psychoanalyst Richard Wollheim describes our desperate attempts to cling on to being:

> Death is the great enemy not merely because it deprives us of all the future things we might do, and all the pleasures we might experience. It takes away the ability to experience anything at all, ever. It puts an end to our being... it deprives us of phenomenology, and, having once tasted phenomenology, we develop a longing for it which we cannot give up.
>
> (Wollheim, 1984, p. 269)

Avoidance of death anxiety

It is this clinging on to our "being" that makes us go to great lengths, consciously or non-consciously, to avoid thinking about our death and experiencing the associated anxiety. A void in someone's life may be a sign of an incohesive sense of self (Hargaden & Sills, 2002), but we need to consider also that it may be a fear of the time that they will not have a self at all. As well as attempts to receive love, acceptance, or respect, we can think of some script and driver behaviour as a defence against death, a frantic attempt to gain control of our lives, to keep on existing and to drown out the unwanted realisation of our impending non-existence. We become immersed in work (or writing books about existence!), a quest for power or control, our families, our social life or hobbies, religion, sex, symbiotic relationships, or over-caring, or we keep "trying" or "hurrying" or "being strong". If we can just be perfect or please others, *then* we can "be" and will not have to experience the anxiety of our non-existence. At its extreme, this presents itself in anxiety disorders, panic disorders, post-traumatic stress disorder, obsessive-compulsive disorders, phobias, addictions, and irrational beliefs and fears.

Yalom (1980) also suggests that people deny death by becoming the ultimate rescuer (the external hero who saves other people from death) or through a belief in their own "specialness" and narcissistic inviolability (the internal hero who believes they are so special they would not be allowed to die). Becker (1973) describes some people believing that the rules of death will no longer apply to them if they can be "heroic", or attempting to overcome death by creating something that will live beyond their death (such as Freud's investment in psychoanalysis). A faith in the existence of an external ultimate rescuer (God, a Higher Being, or the perfect partner) can also "protect" people from the reality of death. Many cultures believe that an ancestor still exists as long as they are remembered, which can be at the root of attempts to become famous or influential, leave a legacy, or perpetuate ourselves through having children or funding a project. If we can still be remembered, we can symbolically never die.

Much good can come from these strivings if the aim is to further humanity, but there will always be something lost if we do not use the awareness of death to help us live fully in the present. Some people circumvent living altogether. They avoid investing in relationships, careers, vocations, or hobbies, believing that if they do not really live, they will not really die. Or as they start facing the reality of their mortality or the awareness that much of life has already been lived (particularly in midlife or after a bereavement, major loss, or threat to life), an ensuing life crisis might lead to sudden life changes. Some affairs in long-term relationships, particularly with much younger partners, can provide an illusion that adult life has started again and enable a fleeting escape from the reality of a life half over. Risky behaviour can also be a way of defying death and confirming aliveness; many adolescents or young adults in particular counteract the emerging realisation of mortality through risk-taking (Spinelli, 2015; Yalom, 1980). When my son was a teenager, he used to deliberately tell me he was going off to do something risky, leaving me with the fear of his death so that he could go off and experiment, feel alive, and have (his idea of) fun! Alternatively, some people avoid risk at any cost to avoid uncertainty, the unknown, and the unforeseen. Otto Rank described the neurotic as one "who refused the loan (life) in order to avoid the payment of the debt (death)" (Rank, 1945, p. 126).

Our spiritual and religious beliefs and socio-cultural heritage influence our response to death. Some cultures with a greater spiritual awareness face death more directly and have an underlying comfort in a more expansive spiritual meaning of life and death, a sense of being part of the universe in an eternal circle of life, or beliefs in an afterlife or reincarnation. Death anxiety can be pacified by religious beliefs which offer certainty of continued existence after death and a comfort of being reunited with loved ones in an afterlife. On the other hand, these beliefs can create more anxiety if there is a fear of judgement by a Higher Being or the possibility of eternal separation from non-believing loved ones. There can also be a great deal of guilt, shame, and impasse if the religious person still fears death or the process of dying, despite the promises of their faith. I have been to several funerals where the focus on a celebration of life or the anticipation of eternal life has discounted the reality of the grief of the present death. In doing so, we also deny facing the reality that one day the person in the coffin will be us.

The risks and consequences of denying death

Rollo May said: "The price for denying death is undefined anxiety, self-alien-ation. To completely understand himself, man must confront death, and become aware of personal death" (May, 1961, p. 65). From earliest childhood I suffered from separation anxiety, resisting any kind of separation from my mum. I would hide letters from school about residential trips in case she encouraged me to go, would avoid sleepovers at friends' houses, and suffered from a lingering and excruciating abandonment depression at university. To avoid the terror of aloneness, I became enmeshed in romantic relationships as a young teen, and married at 23. Being alone in the world felt like a threat to my survival, yet nobody knew the extent of my pain and the constant churning in the pit of my stomach that I felt when considering an accident or illness befalling my mother, and, from adolescence, my partner. Because I did not feel able to talk to my family about my fears and anxieties, I did not real-ise that I was anxious about death. As Boss suggested: "People who are most afraid of *death* are those who have the greatest anxiety about *life*" (Boss, 1979, p. 112; original emphasis). My death anxiety was making me wither away; I was failing to thrive in life, performing well academically but men-tally, emotionally, and spiritually in torment and unable to flourish. Looking back, I did not realise that this was not how many other people experienced life. In not being able to face and tolerate death, I was becoming discon-nected and alienated from my core authentic self, others, and the world. I was alienated from life. It was not until I started relationship therapy in my 30s that the blinkers were removed and I saw more clearly the restrictive prison in which my death anxiety was holding me captive. This was the beginning of a long journey into confronting more fully both death and life, first in under-standing the psychodynamics of the childhood experiences that had led to my separation anxiety, and later in facing the challenging realities and ten-sions of relating, being, death, and human existence. With the companion-ship and involved presence of my therapists and supervisors on this painful yet soulfully enlivening journey, I gradually learnt to face death without being overwhelmed or dominated by it, and to live more fully, vitally, and courageously. As Jean-Jacques Rousseau (cited in van Deurzen & Adams, 2016, p. 140) describes: "We are born, so to speak, twice over; born into exist-ence, and born into life; born a human being, and born a man". Facing death in the presence of an engaged other was helping me finally become an enliv-ened woman.

Danica

My struggles with death anxiety better equipped me to be alongside Danica in hers. She came to see me with severe anxiety that left her largely unable to leave her home following the traumatic death of her eldest sister. Growing up, her sister had been her main attachment figure throughout an abusive and neglectful childhood and adolescence. Death had been ever-present in her family yet had never been spoken about. Her mother had deadened herself through abuse of alcohol and prescribed medication; her father was a well-known and respected public figure who presented externally as a devoted family man but saved his deathly, violent, and destructive tendencies for Danica in the confines of the family home. Danica psychically killed off parts of herself in order to survive, and the death of her sister stirred old wounds and such a sense of grief, helplessness, uncertainty, terror, and lack of control that anxiety became the only way she could manage these archaic split-off ego states. She handled her anxiety by counting in threes and, when particularly acute, hiding in a safe, coffin-sized space under her bed. She found solace in photography and I encouraged her to take photos that expressed her anxiety and despair. Bringing them to me (always in threes), she communicated her deadened parts of self, and her repressed and unsupported history with death. The destructiveness of "mortido" was a regular theme: an animal's skull, a wrecked boat on the shore, an overgrown graveyard, a tree hit by lightning, an abandoned and vandalised building, the guts of roadkill. As we talked about them, we journeyed into the dark depths of Danica's soul and gradually wove together the broken and fragmented threads of death into the tapestry of Danica's life. Together, we found words to make meaning and speak of the terror of death and the abandonment by her mother in her early life, her fear of her own death from her father's violence, the desire for his destruction, the traumatic experiences of her sister dying through medical neglect, as well as her present profound dread of her partner dying that left her waking in a panic most nights to check whether they were still breathing.

Over time, Danica's anxiety faded, replaced by a more energetic liveliness and a simmering unexpressed rage, particularly towards her father who had died eight years' previously. Rather than sadness and grief, his death had provided relief for Danica, and acknowledging and validating this relief seemed to loosen some of the ties to her dead father. When her mother became terminally ill several years into our therapy, she was also able to more fully express her rage. As so often happens when members of our original family are ill or die, old familial existential tensions and struggles emerged around control, power, safety, care, love and hate, conflict, competition, envy, and uncertainty. Danica lived in a different country from her surviving family, and Danica's sister became increasingly cruel and controlling towards Danica, restricting her access to their dying mother and blocking all contact with her. I felt powerless in the face of the sadism and desperately wanted to escape it, yet Danica required me to be in the disturbance and the unresolvable intrapsychic and interpersonal tension with her. She alternated between raging at her sister, at her parents, at herself, at the universe, and she needed me to feel it with her, to help her learn to tolerate her helplessness, to express yet contain her rage, and provide the support that she had lacked in her childhood experiences of sadistic and cruel control. Week after week I listened to and experienced in my body her feelings of helplessness, injustice, anger, hatred towards her sister, and her fear, love, sadness, and grief. It was messy, painful, and distressing work; I left each session deeply disturbed, enraged and immersed in hateful and sadistic feelings. I think I could have killed her sister. Going with her into my own capacity for sadism, yet containing it, enabled her to acknowledge and express her own. Despite being in the midst of death, Danica became enlivened. One session she brought a single photo, and I noticed it was no longer one of three. Had Danica individuated from being "one of three" in her family? It was of a seedling, a strikingly different sign of life, and I commented on it emerging out of a field of mud. "Oh, it's not mud," she said, "it's cow shit. I loved that growth was coming out of the shit".

Danica was integrating the polarities of life and death. As Yalom states: "Life and death are interdependent; they exist simultaneously, not consecutively; death whirs continuously beneath the membrane of life and exerts a vast influence upon experience and conduct" (Yalom, 1980, p. 29). We cannot have death without life and we cannot have an authentic life without an awareness and experience of death and destructiveness. We cannot have growth without shit. In facing death, destructiveness, grief, loss, and change, we are able to live life more fully, know our true self, make more meaningful life choices and feel like we are truly living: "it is only in the face of death that man's self is born" (Saint Augustine, cited in Yalom, 1980, p. 30).

The benefits of facing death

Mindful, vibrant, and authentic living

It is a paradox that the physicality of death *destroys* life, but the facing of death *saves* life. To truly embrace our *being*, the reality of our *non-being* must be faced (Tillich, 1952). Embracing death and its associated terror and grief enables us to become less anxious and fearful, have greater compassion, love and empathy, increased calmness and centredness, gain a new awareness of what is truly important in life, and enable the joys and pains of life to be appreciated and experienced more intently, vibrantly and passionately. Heidegger (1927/2010) said that the awareness of our personal death spurs us to shift from a state of forgetfulness of being, where we immerse ourselves in the everyday diversions of life, to a state of mindfulness and awareness of being, to marvel not about the *way* things are but *that* they are. The night my friend died, I looked out of the curtains at 3am and was overcome with the beauty of a black velvet sky illuminated by a perfectly vivid crescent moon framing the brightest star I had ever seen. Never for me had the "evening star", a symbol of the ending of the day, been so meaningful. The knowledge that my friend would not be able to witness this, or indeed anything, ever again, made me feel both despairing at the finite nature of life, and increasingly determined that I would soak up moments like these while I still could. As Berne described in a moment of here-and-now existential awareness: "Knowing that the trees will still be there after he dies, so [wanting] to experience them now with as much poignancy as possible" (Berne, 1964, pp. 159–160).

Tolerating existential tensions

"Boundary" or "limit" situations in life like death, loss, or endings in therapy and consultation can help jolt us out of the psychic numbing or anxiety of everyday inauthentic existence into mindful and authentic living (Jaspers, 1925/1960). But this comes with an unsolvable existential impasse: the reality of mortality (and its associated existential themes of isolation, responsibility, freedom, and meaning) versus our intense desire to avoid death. Rather than being stuck on either end of the continuum of life and death, an abundant existence accepts the constant ebb and flow between the two as our experiences and stages of life change. We can face death head on but are not consumed or overwhelmed by it.

When her mum died, Danica made me a gift of appreciation – a beautiful wooden star. She couldn't have known how evocative this was for me of my friend's death, yet she knew on a spiritual level that we were both facing the "evening star" of death together. Interestingly, the "evening star" is also known as the "morning star", a symbol of both endings and beginnings, death and life. Unlike her childhood and early adult experiences of death, Danica was now able to hold on to the morning as well as the evening, life at the same time as death. She was able to face her authentic, disturbing, and painful feelings as well as get love and support from me, her partner, friends, colleagues, hobbies, and her humour. The meaning, spiritual connection, and fulfilment this gave her was the "growth from the shit" that enabled her to better tolerate the existential tension between life and death. She did not have to hide under the bed any more.

Working with death and endings

Facing our own death anxiety

We cannot help our clients face the terror of death if we have not reconciled with death ourselves. Yalom (1980) argues that, "Frequently the denial of the therapist silently colludes with that of the patient. The therapist no less than the patient must confront death and be anxious in the face of it" (Yalom, 1980, pp. 204–205). Mothersole suggests that if we fail to confront our own mortality, "we collude in keeping the lid on a can of worms that may be of profound therapeutic importance to our clients" (Mothersole, 1996, p. 157), and suggests that "no-self-harm contracts" (or closing escape hatches) may play a role in "keeping the lid on" so that both parties can avoid the feared issue. I notice that many people find it easier to first face their anxiety about others dying before confronting their own death, and it is often not until we are faced with a significant boundary situation around death, life, and loss that the enormity of our own final ending surfaces. When my marriage ended after 23 years, the immense loss triggered evocative dreams and nightmares about death. I would wake in the night gripped with terror that I was dying, with a sense of an evil presence in my room, or with an acute anxiety that because I had not done something then I now had to die. In my waking life I would have moments of acute panic that I would one day be gone from the world and would not find out what happened in the remainder of my children's lives. The truth was that I *was* dying; my old married, enmeshed self that had never known adult singleness and individuation was dead. My life with a united family unit was over; my dreams and expectations of my own and my family's future were shattered. I genuinely didn't know whether I could survive on my own and as a single parent, and the uncertainty of my new self and unwanted future life was terrifying. Bearing the terror through the help of those who accompanied me through the valley of death, gradually discovering and shaping my new self, and learning to integrate and even admire the scars helped me move from reflectively troubling to reflectively accepted change.

Talking about death

We should not wait for such a crisis to explore our feelings about death; we need to talk about our death and destructiveness in our own supervision, consultation, personal therapy, training, and spiritual accompaniment. If we are to travel with our clients and supervisees as fellow explorer and guide on their journey to the depths, we have a responsibility to first do a reconnaissance of the expedition. Often people circumvent death because it has always been avoided in their family of origin and/or culture. Coming to terms with the concept of death is a major developmental task of every child, but many people in a Western culture, particularly, have had death ignored, brushed under the carpet, and sanitised. Sometimes this has been about protectiveness, considering it inappropriate for children to be exposed to the "nastiness" of death, but instead the child is left isolated, confused, and scared. As a child, my beloved cat was killed by a car and I was left with a neighbour while my parents took her body to the vet. A child in my class died, and another friend's mother was later killed in a car accident, but it was not spoken about and no real explanation was given about death and grieving. Being alone with my mind's fantasies around death simply served to exacerbate my separation anxiety. Some clients were never spoken to about the death of a parent, were not taken to their parent's or sibling's funeral, or had a parent quickly remarry and remove from the house all traces of their deceased parent. One client was not told that their sibling's illness was terminal until they came home from school and they had already been taken to the morgue. The implicit message in all these situations was that death should not be talked about, and each child was left alone with intolerable grief, fear, and terror; a paradoxical awareness of both the inevitability and yet the "unmentionability" of death. I think we need to take responsibility for bringing up the subject of death with clients, supervisees, and trainees and for talking to our clients about their first experiences of death: how they first became aware of it, who they discussed it with, how their families, schools, and adults in their life coped with our clients' questions and fears about death. In doing so we make it "mentionable" and break the taboo; our clients can hear on a profound level that we are willing to be their deep-sea diving partner in their exploration and increasing toleration of their terror of death.

Paying attention to dreams and symbolism

The dreams of clients or practitioner are often a precious route to talking about the unconscious and non-conscious feelings, fantasies, and experiences around death and destructiveness. "Fear of death exists at every level of awareness – from the most conscious, superficial, intellectualized levels to the realm of deepest unconsciousness" (Yalom, 1980, p. 204). I invite my clients, supervisees, and trainees to explore with me their thoughts, feelings, and fantasies around their dreams and the possible messages that lie within them. Often at their root are existential themes around ending and their attitudes and beliefs about death, life, birth, change, transformation, sex, and the erotic. The interdependence of life and death make dreams with the theme of death, birth, and sex especially prevalent around endings. Death is in sight from the moment of birth, and the new life that emerges from the vitality of sex is the antithesis of death: "reproduction is the essential way of counteracting death" (Klein, 1948, pp. 114–123). When my friend died, I dreamt about a friend from my teenage years who had died some years earlier before being able to have children. In my dream I was delighted to see her alive again, breast-feeding a baby, accompanied by the vicar who had married me. I think it vividly illustrated my struggle with accepting my friend's death, as well as perhaps the remnants of loss surrounding the death of my marriage, and my continual striving for life and vitality amidst the endings.

During the last weekend of a four-year training, one of my students dreamt that she was heavily pregnant and her waters broke. Exploring the feelings in the dream helped her express her excitement, fear, and anticipation at the ending of our group and the transition from training into qualification. Another dreamt about having a sexual relationship with me, sex sometimes being an attempt to beat death by affirming life and vitality, and an endeavour to assuage individuation and death anxiety through merger. Our dialogue about his dream helped him celebrate the vitality of our experiences together, as well as the loss of me and the group, and the fear of "going out there alone".

Confronting endings and boundary situations

All boundary situations and endings in therapy will have some implicit link to death, echoing the human condition. Endings are implicit in the relationship from the start of therapy, just as every new relationship will end one day. Like Berne (1966), I hold the ending in mind from the beginning by making this explicit in the assessment session and outlining a preferable ending process in my written contract. I pay particular attention to investigating issues emerging around boundaries: contracting, payment, the beginning and ending of sessions, missed appointments, and the start and end of the therapeutic or consultative relationship. Supervisees sometimes find it difficult to challenge these boundary situations, framing it as a fear of confrontation. I believe it is sometimes more specifically about a fear of confrontation with death. We have a responsibility to be aware of our own relationship and tensions with endings so that we do not unconsciously collude with our clients in avoiding an ending. I recently marked a psychotherapy MSc dissertation that had no mention of endings at all, and each case example came to a sudden and abrupt close, leaving me feeling incomplete and unsatiated at the suddenness of the "cutting off". Endings were being avoided, and I wondered about the candidate's history with their own endings, their own relationship with life and death, as well as their clients' and what was left incomplete in their therapy and thus in their experience of integration of life and death.

We need to confront the defensive avoidance strategies around endings that are employed by our clients, supervisees, and trainees (as well as ourselves) and help bring into awareness unconscious beliefs, fears, and memories around separation, loss, and death. It can help to watch out for old script issues re-emerging and enactments being played out as the ending approaches, often as a way of trying to gain mastery in a situation that evokes the lack of control we have in death. A defence against death can also materialise in physical or psychological withdrawal (such as missing the last session or the last day of a training course); finding new things to talk about to avoid ending; denigrating the therapist or the therapy so that it becomes easier to separate; focusing on the positives about ending (more time and money), or convincing themselves that it is not really an ending: "I can come back if I need to", "I'll still see you at college" and "we'll all keep in touch even if we're not in the same group anymore".

Offering a new experience of ending

A positive, planned, mutually open and honest ending in the presence of an engaged other, who also expresses authentic feelings about the ending, can be an opportunity for a new relational and learning experience for both client and practitioner. It can also be a necessary confrontation of death. A former student of mine wrote to me recently to thank me for an ending weekend some years previously, where creative exercises and rituals helped the group to explore the existential themes that emerge in endings (Clarkson, 2003): satisfaction and achievement; guilt and regret; anger and disappointment; sadness and nostalgia; fear and trepidation; envy and gratitude; relief and release; anticipation; past losses; existential givens and Jung's archetypal events such as birth, marriage, death. I would also add the erotic and sexuality as an essential aspect of endings. She said that facing fully the depth of feeling about an ending had been profoundly impactful for her and had changed how she faced endings with her clients. She wrote beautifully about helping a terminally ill client move from terror of death to greater acceptance and facing unfinished business, whilst acknowledging and grieving that "business" is never fully finished when we die as there is always more to accomplish, learn, or experience. She said that experiencing me sharing the poignancy and vitality of my loss and grief at the ending of our group, and feel viscerally that she and the group had mattered to me, helped her to have the courage to express to her client her own humanity and pain at their final goodbye. This, in turn, enabled her client to more fully and poignantly experience her own, and to communicate that to her loved ones.

With some clients and supervisees, I reflectively disclosed my bereavement. Of course, such decisions about disclosure are highly personal to both practitioner and client and it may be inappropriate to do so for the protection of either party. We do not want our clients to feel that they have to look after us. Yet enabling them to feel and show empathy for me is also necessary in a mutual (albeit asymmetrical) relationship, and can help them move from "I–It" relating to "I–Thou" relating (Buber, 1923). I also believe it is important for us to communicate the universality of grief and to open up the conversation around death, whilst demonstrating that we can face death whilst not being consumed by it. After talking about my bereavement with a training group a student commented on my ability to move fluently between sadness, laughter, and discussion of theory when facing death, and how this gave her something to aspire to. Disclosure is not always so well-received, of course, and sometimes I get it wrong (see Chapter 4 for a discussion on self-disclosure). But demonstrating my humanity alongside erotic vitality is essential in helping people learn that they can be vulnerable *and* enlivened in the face of death.

A trainee who was impacted by me sharing my vulnerability around death sent me a podcast about grief that had helped her in hers. Her courage and the mutuality of humanity was immensely touching. I was also moved by the vulnerability of the radio presenter, who powerfully shared his profound grief at the loss of his sister in the hope this would help listeners feel less alone in theirs. The calls from listeners and my heartfelt tears confirmed to me the potential in thoughtful disclosure. Mutuality in vulnerability helps us feel connected – tutor, student, presenter, listeners all feeling less alone and enabling us to face the existential givens of life and death with greater courage and authenticity.

Balancing life and death

As I come to the end of this chapter, I confess to having some relief that I can have some respite from immersion in death! Becker (1973) argues that it would be impossible to live in constant conscious awareness of death as this would be too overwhelming and drive people to neurosis or psychosis. I don't think I'm too far away from that! Living with the constant fear of or obsession with death is as equally destructive as living oblivious to the reality of death. Yet as I turn, with some delight, to writing about the erotic, I know that death will never be far behind, for death and the erotic are conjoined. An abundant, intimate, and authentic life embraces death, destruction, and despair, as well as creativity, joy, laughter, excitement, sexuality, and erotic vitality. James Baldwin sums it up beautifully in a passage from "The Fire Next Time", sent to me by a thoughtful student:

> Life is tragic simply because the earth turns and the sun inexorably rises and sets, and one day, for each of us, the sun will go down for the last, last time. Perhaps the whole root of our trouble, the human trouble, is that we will

sacrifice all the beauty of our lives, will imprison ourselves in totems, taboos, crosses, blood sacrifices, steeples, mosques, races, armies, flags, nations, in order to deny the fact of death, the only fact we have. It seems to me that one ought to rejoice in the fact of death – ought to decide, indeed, to **earn** one's death by confronting with passion the conundrum of life.[1]

(Baldwin, 1963/2017, p. 79)

Note

1 James Baldwin, excerpts from *The Fire Next Time*. Copyright © 1962, 1963 by James Baldwin, renewed 1991, 1992 by Gloria Baldwin Karefa-Smart. Reprinted with the permission of The Permissions Company, LLC on behalf of the James Baldwin Estate.

Chapter 13

The erotic life force

Being sexual

The tension between death fear and life fear

It is just as possible to get stuck in the polarity of fear of living as it is the fear of death. Being fully and erotically alive brings death into sharper focus and makes the loss of existence seem even more abhorrent: "The irony of man's condition is that the deepest need is to be free of the anxiety of death and annihilation; but it is life itself which awakens it and so we must shrink from being fully alive" (Becker, 1973, p. 66). Shrinking from both death and erotic aliveness means living in a zombified condition, a state of "psychic numbing"; we come fully into our erotic aliveness when we can tolerate the tension of the inevitable and constant flow between life fear and death fear, vitality and mortality (Rank, 1945). Kierkegaard (cited in May, 1977, p. 38) describes this as the perils of "venturing" and "not venturing": in attempting to individuate, affirm our autonomy, and push ourselves to fulfil our potential, we are brought face-to-face with our fear of life, aloneness, separation, and standing out. We then relinquish our individuation and retreat into the comfort of fusing with another, which evokes the fear of death, stagnation, loss of individuality, not fulfilling our potential, and being dissolved again into the whole. This then propels us to seek aliveness and individuation once again as we venture anew into our erotic life force.

What is "the erotic"?

Plato and the Ancient Greek perspective

There can be confusion about the meaning of the erotic, as contemporary Western culture equates it with sex and often sexualisation and objectification. Sex is one bodily manifestation of a person's sexuality and their erotic life force, but it is not the whole. Eros was a "daimon" in Greek mythology, a creature between divinity and mortality who had a powerful, immortal healing factor. Plato (1993) conceived the erotic as a vehicle for transformation and union with the "Divine", a fundamental life-preserving, creative, and aesthetic

DOI: 10.4324/9781003475217-17

impulse with a sensual element linked to desire that did not necessarily include physical attraction. The word Eros in Ancient Greek meant "love, desire": a sensual, passionate, creative, healing, and spiritual love differentiated from "*storge*" (affection), "*philia*" (friendship), and "*agape*" (charity). In describing these different forms of love, C.S. Lewis (1960/2002) pictured "*eros*" as two people normally face to face, absorbed by each other, which sounds remarkably similar to the love, hate, intimacy, and confrontation of the therapeutic relationship! The erotic in psychotherapy is therefore about relatedness and the aspiration for growth, healing, creativity, recognition, connectedness, and spiritual or transpersonal "I–Thou" (Buber, 1923) encounter. It is also about the drive for wholeness, and integration is not possible without facing the shadow of Eros: Thanatos.

Freud's Thanatos and Eros

Thanatos (Ancient Greek for "death") and Eros were introduced into psychoanalysis by Sigmund Freud (1940/1949, p. 108), described as rival unconscious "primal forces" or drives that motivate human behaviour. Freud saw Eros as the drive of life, love, creativity, self-satisfaction, sexuality, and species preservation, while Thanatos the drive of aggression, sadism, violence, death, and destructiveness. Freud seemed to use "eros" and "libido" interchangeably, originally associating them primarily with sexual urges but later more widely as a general constructive life instinct connected to self-preservation and survival. This was developed further by Jung (1912/2023), who, like Plato, acknowledged the sexual as a fundamental part of the erotic but focused more on the erotic striving for passion, wholeness, psychic relatedness, and interconnection with other sentient beings.

Berne's Mortido and Physis

In transactional analysis (TA), Berne (1972) drew on Freud's life and death drives with his concepts of "mortido" and "physis". He described "mortido" as the death instinct and based his life script theory on Freud's repetition compulsion and mankind's tendency to destructiveness – individually, and in groups, organisations, and nations. He described the human existential tensions between life and death in the form of the "four horsemen of the Apocalypse: war or peace, famine or plenty, pestilence or health, death or life" (Berne, 1972, p. 21), and believed that part of human existence is a capacity for evil that is an inherent aspect of each person's primitive protocol: "The small fascist in every human being is a little torturer who probes for and enjoys the weakness of his victims..." and "[forms] the basis for third-degree 'tissue' games that draw blood" (Berne, 1972, pp. 268–70).

Berne also saw (in each person's protocol) a simultaneous inner drive to health, growth, life, and a need for recognition, which he variously labelled eros (the life force), libido (the sexual instinct, energy, and the need for loving recognition), and physis (a creative life force in the somatic Child that counteracts script) (Clarkson, 1992). Berne described physis as:

> the growth force of nature, which makes organisms evolve into higher forms, embryos develop into adults, sick people get better, and healthy people strive to attain their ideals. Possibly it is only one aspect of inwardly directed libido, but it may be a more basic force than libido itself.
>
> (Berne, 1947/1968, pp. 369–370)

After Berne's death, English (2008) developed further the concept of conflictual unconscious drives in TA, describing Survia (for individual survival – pain, hunger, fear); Passia (for survival of the species – creativity, discoveries, explorations, inventions, risk-taking, playfulness, enthusiasm, pro-creation, and sexuality); and Transcia (for transcendence beyond daily reality – peace and detachment from worldly cares through relaxation, sleep, and spiritual experiences). Like Freud, she described love and aggressiveness as pertaining to all three drives.

Sex and sexuality in TA

In the later years of his life, Berne himself moved from thinking about drives to sex, sexuality and intimacy as an aspect of the erotic and physis (Berne, 1970). It is widely considered, however, that his thinking was extremely limited (Cook, 2022; Karpman, 2010). Cornell is forthright in his critique: "Berne left us with a trite and impoverished literature about sexuality and intimacy" (Cornell, 2009, p. 137), and was rather more complimentary about Steiner's (1986) advocacy for the centrality of sexuality in intimacy and human relations. Other than a focus on sexual abuse, and sexual problems and "dysfunctions", the concept of sexuality as an essential aspect of existence and identity was not fully explored in TA until the 2000s, when a more inclusive, fluid, constructivist, and socio-political perspective to sexuality and identity was advocated, mainly in two special editions of the *Transactional Analysis Journal* (Barnes, 2004; Cornell & Simerly, 2004; Johnson, 2004; Shadbolt, 2004; Cornell, 2009; Shadbolt, 2009; van Beekum, 2009; Blake, 2017; Johnson, 2017; McClean, 2017; Rosario, 2017; Shadbolt, 2017; Rowland & Cornell, 2021).

Relational TA and the erotic transference

At the same time, a relational psychoanalytic perspective to the erotic (Atlas, 2015; Gabbard, 1994; Mann, 1997) was introduced into TA through Hargaden's (2001) case study of an erotic transference and responses from Cornell (2001), Erskine (2001), and Sills (2001). This was further developed by Hargaden & Sills (2002), Kellett (2004), Woods (2005), Cornell (2009), Hargaden (2011), and Little (2018). More recently, TA authors have written about working with the erotic transference in supervision (Hunt & Sills, 2021; Shadbolt, 2021; van Rijn, 2021) and working ethically with erotic transference (Eusden, 2021; van Rijn, 2021). Through these authors, the erotic is now seen in TA as a transferential dynamic that is as much about the psychological as the physical, and its emergence in therapy as a communication about unconscious early child longings and split-off parts of self in Child ego states, in parallel with an unconscious striving for growth and communication of adult sexuality.

Little's (2018) outline of the psychoanalytic perspective to erotic transference and countertransference examines both the defensive and transformational potential of the erotic within psychotherapy. He suggests that both old and new co-created self-other configurations are able to emerge in the erotic transference. Hargaden and Sills (2002) see these configurations in terms of three different domains of transference. The erotic can emerge as an introjective transference, communicating the client's archaic infantile longings (pictured in early Child ego states) and a desire or need to psychically "take in" the therapist. A defensive "eroticized transference" (Blum, 1973) can be experienced in the idolising or denigrating of the therapist, communicating through a projective transference the split and disowned parts of self. This may involve sexualisation, sadomasochism, control, or an avoidance of grief and loss, particularly about the unavailability of the therapist for a real relationship (Maroda, 1999). Possible with both introjective and projective transferences is the therapist's projective identification with the client's earliest disowned sexual, loving, or hateful feelings. Processing for the client what is too unbearable for them to feel for themselves, the therapist gradually feeds back to their client what they are holding to help them to own these cut off parts of self for themselves. Through dialogue, relationship, and the therapist's use of self in the transference, the client is therefore more able to embrace their adult sexuality and transform infantile longings into mature adult love. Crucially, Hargaden (2011) emphasises that the erotic transference is *symbolic* of the child's early longings and the adult's striving for growth, and there is a danger of "acting out" if we concretise as reality our sexual, loving or hateful countertransference.

An existential perspective to the erotic

Being sexual

Of course, the erotic comes with risk of boundary violations for us all because of its seductiveness, excitement and energy. Pope and Bouhoutsos (1986) found that 87% of therapists experience sexual attraction towards their clients (and I would suggest that 13% are discounting on some level!). The moment we are arrogant or naive enough to consider ourselves immune from temptation or the lure of erotic attraction is when we are at risk of harmful transgressions. However, in recognising and revering the powerful unconscious transferential and symbolic processes at play, let us not forget the coexistent existential perspective to the erotic: the healthy, normal, and essential aspect of our human existence that is an inherent part of our search for meaning, passion, and power in life. The erotic and its shadow are not just transferential, it is ever-present from conception to death: attraction, desire, fascination, love, connection, healthy aggression, pleasure at another's bodily presence, being in love, sensual and sexual arousal, age-appropriate sexual acts, as well as the less palatable disgust, repulsion, hate, shame, sadism, malignant aggression, isolation, judgement, and envy. Through attuning to our erotic (and destructive) connections with our clients we can help bring to light the destructiveness of past eroticism and help them metamorphosise into an increasingly vital, creative, sexual and erotic adult human being, whilst acknowledging our universal capacity for destruction. As Cornell (2001) argues:

> It is our willingness to enter the arena of erotic anguish, desire, and delight with our clients that offers them the opportunity to restore the vitality of the body, to leave behind the deadness and distortion of parent/infant eroticism gone bad, and to open up to the world of passionate, adult intimacy and uncertainty.
>
> (Cornell, 2001, p. 239)

For the existentialist, erotic aliveness is indistinguishable from existence and is about "being sexual" (Spinelli, 2015). Our sexuality is the "skeleton" on which all relations with others are hung (Sartre, 1957) and "always present like an atmosphere... Sexuality permeates existence and vice-versa" (Merleau-Ponty, 1962, pp. 168–169). For that reason, Smith-Pickard (2014) prefers to use the term "existential sexuality", which I describe in more detail below. The sexual act is one way we manifest our sexuality and a significant point on the spectrum of existential sexuality, but not the main or only position. The erotic – our sexuality – is therefore in every relationship (albeit sometimes distorted, destructive, or deadened) and if we do not welcome our sexualities and human erotic encounter into the immediacy and intimacy of our consultation rooms, we are negating something of the other's existence. This encounter will involve a swirling energy of unconscious transferential dynamics from the past as well as present-moment conscious and non-conscious adult existential sexuality. I therefore prefer to think of "the erotic" rather than simply "the erotic transference", to account for the multiplicity of transferential, non-transferential, conscious and non-conscious relating. Cornell is perhaps the TA author who has best expressed their interweaving:

> Psychotherapy without attention to sexuality is impoverished. There are few domains of human experience and passion that bring together conscious desire, unconscious motivations, somatic experience, and relationality in the way we can experience this intermingling of forces in sexuality.
>
> (Cornell, 2009, pp. 145–146)

Existential sexuality

Ever-changing identities

So how do we understand existential sexuality? Sexuality is a hard concept to pin down, and perhaps it is not desirable to attempt to do so for this would be reductionist about life and existence. It is deeply personal to each individual, embedded in our cultural and historical context, expressed in individual ways in different relationships and social groupings, and changes over time as we accumulate senses of self throughout our lifetime. Towards the end of my work with a 90-year-old client where we had together explored her identity in late adulthood, I visited her in hospital after a fall. Whilst the other geriatric patients around her looked like they were in God's waiting room, she was enjoying the attentions of the male staff, appreciatively and playfully exclaiming, "there are a lot of nice young men in here!" She was continuing to embrace her sexuality in a way that was accessible to her in the context of her life stage and circumstances, an affirming example of Cornell's description of sexuality as "a refusal to give up on life" (Cornell, 2009, p. 146).

The existential concept of sexuality is not a defining characteristic of an individual but covers desires, practices, relationship statuses, and identities (Milton, 2014). Simpson (2023) suggests that sexuality defines our identity in direct and indirect ways: direct in terms of sexual orientation, gender, attraction, arousal, and sexual behaviours, and indirect in terms of how it influences and is influenced by politics, law, morality, religious beliefs, cultural norms, family dynamics, fashion, art, and all relationships. It is thus not simply dependent on sex or sexual actions, but is coextensive with life and interpersonal engagement (Smith-Pickard, 2014). After presenting a workshop, two of my supervisees independently told me that I had looked beautiful. Somewhat surprised, I enquired what they meant; I did not *feel* objectified (and rather felt warm, connected, and appreciated) but was curious whether, as a woman, I was being seen for my looks rather than my mind. On the contrary, their perspective of beauty was holistic and expansive rather than reductionist. They described an appreciation of the integration of body, mind, and spirit, the "aesthetics of being sexual" (Spinelli, 2014, p. 53) that was expressed through my physical appearance and how I held my body, as well as the passion, authenticity, and playfulness I exuded when talking about a topic I truly believed in. I'm sure they wouldn't have considered me so beautiful that morning when, rather less passionately, I put the bins out! Yet in that moment the wider meaning of beauty – an erotic aliveness and sexuality – was recognised, appreciated, and expressed.

Validation of existence

I am just as curious if I *don't* experience a client as beautiful, attractive or with an erotic presence in some way, as "personal existence always has a sexual meaning or colouring" (Madison, 1981, pp. 47–48). What has happened to their erotic liveliness? Through our sexuality and erotic vitality, we get our existence validated, and a lack of sexual attraction (which does not necessarily mean the desire to have sex) can feel like a negation of one's whole being. When love, desire, sexuality, and healthy aggression has been rejected or shut down in early life because of the caregiver's own repression or denial, the repeated and traumatic non-verbal messages about the denial or rejection of their existence or being-in-the-world can impact negatively a person's perception of their sexuality and their vital, erotic existence. This is often communicated through a deadening of desire in the therapeutic relationship. Too often, the therapist contributes to this deadening out of fear or anxiety of their own emerging sexual feelings. They can use theory to attribute the desire in the room to the client's transference, whilst disavowing their own bodily responses and the very real sexual feelings that are being evoked for them in relationship with another sexual being. As therapists, if we are to help our clients move from death into life, we need to be open to their bodily impact on us and to embrace the possibility of mutuality of desire.

Erotic desire

It is through mutual desire that we awaken each other to our authentic self and our inter-relational beings: in desiring you, I make a difference to you in validating your existence through my embodied presence. Being able to make a difference enables me to know that I am. When you desire me, you communicate that you see me for who I am, you acknowledge and confirm my existence through your embodied presence. "Desire is an expression of a yearning to know ourselves through the other" (Pearce, 2011, p. 238), and being sexual evokes desire. It enables us to seduce, attract, or enchant the other, capturing their attention and consciousness. We learnt to do this in different ways from childhood, sometimes in a distorted manner because it was the only way of having our existence validated, but often in creative, charismatic, magnetic, and ingenious approaches that invite reciprocal responses from the other. The emergence of seduction and desire for client and practitioner in the therapy or consulting room is therefore not necessarily pathological, but can be a primal and human need for each other. Of course, out of awareness our seduction can also be destructive, manipulative, and objectifying. Non-conscious seduction risks the use of our clients for our own narcissistic gains. Rather than pathologise our ability to seduce, however, we need trusted others (therapists, supervisors, consultants, colleagues) to help bring our seductiveness into consciousness and entice it out of the shadows into the light. We can then help our clients do the same, enabling us to healthily seduce each other through the expression of our sexuality and thereby validating each other's erotic existence.

Working with the erotic

Shame and the mutuality of self-disclosure

Because of the capacity for transgression and the evocation of shame, therapist self-disclosure around the erotic is particularly contentious. I discuss self-disclosure further in Chapter 4, but in no other area is it more important to remember the power of our role and the asymmetry of the therapeutic relationship. I remember with embarrassment my first foray into talking about the erotic with a client, energised and passionate after a weekend's training. I was a little too eager to talk about his subtle flirting, and the look of horror and mortification on that poor man's face is still engraved on my mind two decades later! We sat together red-faced in a pool of shame and embarrassment, both completely at a loss with where to go next, and our relationship never fully recovered. I believe I had pathologised him in enquiring about and confronting *his* transference onto me (rather than accepting myself as part of the dynamic). I had neither acknowledged my considerable power and the potential for shame, nor had fully considered the mutuality of the erotic encounter.

Whilst never losing sight of the asymmetry of the therapeutic relationship, I now see mutuality as the most important aspect of working with the erotic: mutual influence, mutual recognition, mutual accommodation, mutual negotiation, and mutual change (Aron, 2008). It is the courage of mutuality that ensures humility and the offering of our vulnerable humanity which can counteract shame. Mutuality normalises the erotic and cultivates an atmosphere where sexual feelings and desires can be openly talked about with acceptance and curiosity rather than judgement or fear. It is mutuality that enables us to account for our contribution to a heightened erotic tension, rather than using the notion of countertransference to avoid taking responsibility for our own experiences, feelings and attraction (O'Shea, 2000). Spinelli (1994) invites a mutuality in relationship by being thoughtfully and reflectively open and authentic with our desire and sexual feelings:

> ...rather than seek to deny or suppress such feelings, or, alternatively, to "transform" them or minimise their impact by invoking such terms as "counter-transference", therapists might do better to *acknowledge* them as being present in their experience of, and relationship with, their client.
>
> (Spinelli, 1994, p. 114, original emphasis)

Whilst this often involves acknowledging these feelings to ourselves and our supervisor and enjoying the vitality of the erotic field rather than overt self-disclosure (Dimen, 2024), existential psychotherapy research has shown that reflexive self-disclosure of sexual feelings, attraction or enjoyment of our clients can foster honesty, authenticity, and personal responsibility (Marshall & Milton, 2014). Importantly, it can also demonstrate to the client that sexuality and desire is not something of which to be ashamed. For where there is intimacy, excitement, and desire, feelings of shame, fear, anxiety, and judgement are never far behind. We need to learn to manage our own affect and emotional responses to the erotic so that we can offer containment to our clients in our dialogue. In doing so, we can help them make meaning of the desire (and shame), rather than focus on the attraction itself (Berry, 2014).

Oliver

This meaning-making process was significant in my work with Oliver. Our sessions were becoming increasingly stuck because of what felt like an unspoken and distracting attraction between us. After considerable reflection in supervision, I broached the subject with Oliver in an attempt to loosen the impasse and make meaning together. I did not anticipate Oliver's response. Simply mentioning desire evoked such a shame response in him that he shut me down quite brutally, leaving me feeling bruised and shame-ridden myself. Trying to rescue the situation – and myself – I defensively attempted to make meaning by interpreting our relating as transferential, which left him feeling pathologised and shamed once more and he went further into defence. What had started as an attempt at deeper connection resulted in a disturbing dynamic of alternating positions of control and shame, where both of us felt objectified by the other. I was left wishing that I had kept the lid firmly on the erotic can of worms! However, our relationship had solid foundations, and we slowly (and sometimes agonisingly) used our rupture to explore our co-created power, gender, and sexual dynamics. We began to understand the interplay between our competing desires for withdrawal and connection, and our interlocking protocol-level fears of abandonment and engulfment. We endured our shame enough to investigate how dominance, submission, control, and desire played out between us – themes which Sartre (1943/1956) argues are so often at the root of sexual relations. And underneath our defence of control and "malignant aggression" (Fromm, 1974), we uncovered a mutual existential anxiety around uncertainty, impotence, and powerlessness. Our commitment to each other enabled us to survive these disturbing dynamics and experiment with a different "benign aggression" – the potency needed for healthy sexuality which Fromm describes as the ability to move "forwards towards a goal without undue hesitation, doubt or fear" (Fromm, 1974, p. 256). Perhaps most powerfully and movingly, a year after my initial self-disclosure, we were able to vulnerably acknowledge to each other the mutuality of our attraction and care. In becoming able to celebrate respectfully both desiring and being desired we used our power not to destroy or control, but to validate and expand the other's existence.

Risk, reflection, and erotic living

We mitigate the risks associated with self-disclosure and discourse about the erotic with continual reflection about the possible conscious and unconscious dynamics at play: self-reflection, reflection in action, reflection before action, and reflection after action (Aron, 2008). Our supervisors and consultants are our partners-in-reflection and companions-in-play. This is not always a play that is pleasant but one that "represents the freedom and capacity for one to come up against other people and the external world in all its manifestations" (Cornell, 2011, p. 341). Supervision of the existential erotic encounter is thus a co-creative space for mess, mistakes, disturbance, experimentation, fun, fantasies, desire, curiosity, thoughtful risk-taking, and reflective-play. It should offer a mutual, challenging, supportive, and non-judgemental relationship where anything can be talked about and no conversation or emotional response is off-limits; a "vital" relationship in both senses of the word – essential and energised.

Difficulties come when the person in power – supervisor, consultant, trainer, or therapist – is in some form of denial about their sexuality, destructiveness, and erotic vitality, are avoidant of conflict and disturbance, have challenges with celebrating and expressing their own sexuality, or find it hard to notice, embrace, or affirm another's. If the practitioner desperately focuses on providing a "secure base" of a safe, stabilising, nurturing, and predictable relationship rather than the unpredictable, lively, disturbing, uncertain, and challenging "vital base" that the erotic demands (Cornell, 2001, 2009), therapy and supervision risk becoming impotent or even harmful. We need a commitment to reflect deeply on which aspects of vital erotic existence and expression are lacking in our lives, and take the risk to engage with them more fully: our sexuality; sensuality and embodiment; playfulness; power and vulnerability; creativity; intellectuality; emotionality; relationality; spirituality. Living more vitally enables us to hold in mind all aspects of erotic existence when with our clients and supervisees, helping them identify any areas of deadness or drought in their own lives.

Embodiment and sensuality

It is through our bodies and senses that we can discover our vitality. Embodiment is an existential given of life and an "ever-present phenomenon for humans" (Smith-Pickard, 2014, p. 68): we always exist in and through our bodies and "sexual feelings are a constant horizon to our existence" (Smith-Pickard, 2014, p. 68). It is through our bodies that we can express sexual desire and through embodied encounter that our erotic vitality and sexuality can be revealed and impressed upon the other. Through being sexual, we capture the other's awareness, and both of us receive the otherness and sexuality of the other person as a bodily felt experience even without physical touch. A movement of our body or chair to come closer or further away is a powerful communication. That is not to say that touch is prohibited in the therapy room; far from it, as touch is vital to life and humanity and therefore sometimes helpful in the therapeutic encounter. Sensitive and reflective touch with the client's permission, and enquiry into how they experienced the touch, can provide a route into their erotic, sexual, and spiritual being and associated feelings of love, desire, hate, and disgust.

Recognising sensations in our own bodies can also help us guide our clients in becoming more conscious of their own. Barrow (2018) talks about this as being more aware of *being* a body, not simply having a body. What is it that transfixes us and draws in our being? What arouses, excites, soothes, or disturbs our bodies? Being sexual and experiencing erotic aliveness is dependent on us recognising, appreciating, and expressing beauty, darkness, and disturbance through our senses: sight (art, film, colour, nature, animals, a person's body), hearing (music, the breeze or violent wind, thunder, birds singing, a purring or yowling cat, waves lapping on the stony shore or crashing on rocks), taste (delicious or repulsive food, fine wine, soured milk, a sweet blackberry picked from the brambles), touch (massage, holding hands, banging our shins or stubbing our toe, hugs, masturbation, patting a dog, stroking a cat, being scratched by a cat, silk clothing or a velvet cushion, a rough sack, the rays of the sun, sand on our toes, cold water, a warm bath, squelchy mud, a thorny rose), and smell (a new-born baby, perfume, flowers, cut grass, fresh bread baking, faeces, vomit, rotten food). When an experience combines several senses, and a contrast between delight and disgust, the erotic and sexual vitality can be particularly intense.

Just as our existence is unique to each individual, so is our embodied experience. What delights me may disgust you. We benefit from recognising our similarities and differences in how we experience the light and shade of our own sexuality and that of another. For me, it is when I feel a shivering and tingling in my body, a warmth rising and falling, goose bumps all over my body, or a physical repulsion, tension in my shoulders, churning stomach, or nausea. When I can't keep my eyes off someone, feel transfixed or entranced or repulsed by their smell, their face, their voice, the movement of their body, their eyes or smile. When I feel a sexual arousal of my genitals and erogenous zones, a desire to touch or to be touched (sensually or sexually), or a strong repulsion at the idea of doing so. When I experience butterflies or a roller-coaster in my stomach, find myself smiling or glowering with my eyes, clenching my jaw or grinding my teeth, or feeling a bodily or facial glow, an intense feeling of love or being in love, sweating palms, a redness rising in my cheeks, or a vigorous bodily heat or frozenness of anger, hatred, or fear. Silently noticing the mutual impact of our embodied presence on each other, and sometimes dialoguing about it, we can both hear the silent communication of early relational trauma and protocol that is held in the body, whilst also offering an embodied route into greater freedom, aliveness, and erotic and sexual vitality in their present existence (Cornell & Landaiche, 2006; Novak, 2016).

Authenticity in sexuality

We need to ensure that we do not reduce our clients' lived experiences of their sexuality to our fixed perspective or frame of reference. We want to help them become aware of their own unique authentic beliefs and values about being sexual and how they might have been living inauthentically because of their sociocultural context and their familial and cultural norms. How do they now want to express their sexuality?

Damien

I struggled to connect erotically with Damien for several months, his presence pallid and his speech dirge-like. He didn't seem to know why he had come, he just wanted to be with me, yet he also wasn't giving me much to go on. Through talking about our struggle, he identified a black void in his life that was manifesting in the room, but he couldn't picture it, identify it, or connect with it. I suggested he create something that expressed it and he showed a glimmer of enthusiasm as he left the session. The following week he returned, having created a sculpture using a block of wood and a chainsaw. One side was flat and completely black, the other violently hacked to pieces by the power tool. The horror film *Texas Chainsaw Massacre* wouldn't leave my mind. "I've been living a lie," he announced breathlessly and with a vitality I hadn't yet experienced in him. "I've been sexually attracted to men for 40 years and I haven't told anyone, not even my wife". The main character in the film was a cannibal who wore a mask of human skin; Damien's creativity opened up a passage for us to go behind the 40-year-old mask into his authentic erotic and sexual being and his associated shame, murderous rage, and sadomasochistic urges. He had been "eating himself up" with guilt and shame and he did not have to do this any longer. He could decide for himself how he wanted to be authentic in his sexuality, which in turn presented him with different uncertainties and existential angst at having freedom and choice, with corresponding responsibility for the impact of his decisions on his wife and children. "Being sexual existentially takes us away from the certainty and security of an imposed 'I am…' and places us in the uncertain terrain of 'I am being…'" (Spinelli, 2014, p. 57). Authenticity is not always the easy option, but it surely is a more life-giving alternative than self-cannibalisation.

Sessy

Creativity

Sessy was so deadened and depressed in our first session that she sat in my therapy room lifeless and expressionless, unable to look me in the eye. Yet I experienced a vitality in me that desperately wanted to connect with her. I found myself making gentle but slightly challenging jokes and was met with a flicker of a smile which hooked me in for more, seducing me into validating her existence. Sessy later told me that my humour confirmed I was the right person for her; it was a glimmer of light that her innate playfulness could be resurrected. Our immediate, spiritual, and erotic connection enabled her creativity to unfold. She brought to the session a picture she had drawn of an impenetrable door barricaded by firmly nailed planks and sporting a "No Entry" sign. "We are not going there," was the strong communication. She was throwing down the gauntlet; thankfully, I could match her strong will! She was evoking in me a desire and burning curiosity – to know Sessy, to find out what was behind that door, to bring to life her deadened parts. Week after week Sessy brought to session evocative, moving and disturbing pictures, a non-verbal communication of her deep distress and a challenge to come and find her, yet also a threat of "don't you dare". Her pictures were covered with staring eyes, as if in a horror movie, and she admitted that my gaze was too intense for her. I needed to up my game and think more creatively. We shared a love of nature so I suggested we experiment with side-by-side outdoor sessions, which made Sessy light up. Despite her obvious vulnerability, it felt that Sessy was firmly in control.

Disturbance

Being outside shifted something for Sessy, reporting feeling more in her body. Her pictures became increasingly complex, disturbing, and violent. Death, destruction, torture, a black void, and a blue, lifeless heart were common themes as she started to let me through the barricaded door and communicated her destructive urges towards herself and others, including me. She drew a pirate ship with a skull and crossbones, and started calling me "Captain Cook", a witty but slightly alarming twist of my name, bearing in mind that Captain Cook had been killed by the indigenous Hawaiians he had been attempting to colonise. "If I'm Captain, what's your current role on the ship? First Mate?" I asked, nervously attempting to balance the power. "Deckhand," was her speedy reply. Once again, I attempted to redress the power differential, feeling uneasy on my pedestal and my potential for colonisation. "One day you'll take over captaining this ship and I'll alight at the dock and wave you off on your next voyage". "Oh no," she responded with a seemingly sadistic enjoyment, "you'll be walking the plank". I felt a shiver down my spine at her ruthlessness and cruelty, simultaneously disturbed and excited at the depths we were traversing.

Power and vulnerability

Despite me being "Captain", Sessy was clearly in control of our ship. She determined how we spent each session and gave me meticulous-ly-prepared "homework". I found myself uncharacteristically submis-sively completing it for fear of disappointing her. I fantasised about the film *The Mutiny on the Bounty*, when disaffected crewmen seized control of their ship from their Captain. Was I also going to be set adrift? Despite this, there was a touching vulnerability, affection, and sponta-neity between us. Sessy had a lively curiosity and really wanted to know me, which seduced me into self-disclosing far more than usual. I asked her what that was like. "I need to know you're human so I can trust you", she said. The mutuality of our vulnerability helped reduce my power, which seemed to enable Sessy to trust, perhaps because she felt in control.

Play

With greater mutuality came playfulness. We sparred off each other intellectually, our inquisitive minds challenging each other's frame of reference and inspiring further creativity. Thinking is often dismissed erroneously as a defence against feeling when it can also be a playful-ness of erotic passion and energy which creates something new. As we played, we laughed together more, sometimes a black humour and often until our bellies hurt. Rather than colluding with a gallows or gamy laugh, or being a "Witch Parent" laugh of derision or defeat (Berne, 1972), this usually felt like an intimate, erotic, affectionate and challenging shared humour. We laughed to repair ruptures, confront script, and when gaining insight (Berne, 1972), and Sessy reported that laughing in the face of adversity helped her tolerate the anxieties, tensions and uncertainties of life. Laughter is essential to our erotic life force from birth to death. It is part of our "indomitable core of self" (Erikson, 1997), an energy that helps me connect with both my three-month-old great-niece and my 90-year-old mum with dementia, and through laughter Sessy started coming back to life.

Laughter also connects us to our shadow. Cornell (2014, citing Winnicott, 1971) suggests that the excitement and precariousness of play and intimacy is because of the fusion of constructive and destructive forces – aggression with sexuality – that permeates all our lives and can be integrated through play and creativity. For Sessy and me, the fusion of constructive and destructive forces came through our mutual teasing. We were both the youngest child in large families and teasing was familiar, affectionate, flirtatious, and seductive. There was also a risky, ever-present threat of aggression, like two cats who start play-fighting but end up with claws, teeth and fur flying! The teeth and claws came out when I began resisting Sessy's control. She brought a picture to a session, with a script for me to read, and I declined. The atmosphere felt alive with tension and danger. Her picture of my therapy room was evocative of the stand-off. On my chair sat a ginger cat, on hers was a pigeon, the same size as the cat and meeting the cat's stare equally intensely. It reminded me of my cat sizing up the pigeons in the garden, desperately wanting to hunt them but not daring to because of being pecked ferociously! Was I about to walk the plank? Or make her walk mine? I had often shared with Sessy when her questions made me feel like I was being trapped, and in her picture a sign on the wall read, "This is not a trap". Yet the rug on the floor between us looked remarkably like a trap door and I felt it opening up between us. I experienced the tone of Sessy's teasing subtly turning to one of derision and intimidation rather than affection and, feeling wounded, I told her that the vulnerabilities I had shared now felt like a nuclear weapon deterrent she was threatening to use against me. This wounded and shamed her, the trap door opened and we both fell forcibly out of the pirate ship into shark-infested waters.

Power-over to power-with

Over the next sessions we desperately trod water to keep our heads above the surface as we explored the power, vulnerability, and shame in our relationship. The plank and nuclear weapon analogies began to make sense when she spoke of the sadomasochism of her father who smashed her head against a wall and held a gun to his own head, threatening to pull the trigger in front of her. Her fear and rage surfaced, both with her father and with the oppression and alienation she had experienced as a lesbian growing up in "Bible Belt" America. Our aggressive play gradually shifted from alternating malignant "power-over" sadomasochistic dynamics to a more mutual "power-with" and "power-from-within" (Proctor, 2017), the constructive aggressive power that enables a person to have an effect in the world and is "the capacity to produce change" (Steiner, 1987, p. 102). Foucault argues that such creative power "traverses and produces things, it induces pleasure, forms knowledge, produces discourse. It needs to be considered as a productive network which runs through the whole body, much more than as a negative instance whose function is repression" (Foucault, 1980, p. 119).

Play enabled greater integration of the existential tension between Sessy's creativity and destructiveness, as well as my own. "In play an object can be destroyed and restored; hurt and mended; dirtied and cleaned; killed and brought to life; With the added achievement of ambivalence in place of splitting the object (and self) into good and bad" (Winnicott, 1989, pp. 60–61). When my son was three, he used to play regularly with two imaginary friends until I realised he was only playing with one. When I asked whether the other was, he said sadly, "She died, she was hit by a car"! Through his imaginative play he was making sense of the world, life, death, and loss, his aggressive and destructive urges, and his capacity to restore, love and grieve. Sessy was doing the same with me.

Existential impasses

Sessy's pictures began communicating the ambivalence and existential impasses with which we were tussling. A yellow light piercing the darkness; a dead and rotting carcass of a tree alongside one budding into life; a heart half oxygen-starved blue, half pinking up; the pirate ship half wrecked with tattered sails, the other half bathed in sunlight and vibrant billowing sails. They articulated pleasure and pain, connected-ness and isolation, certainty and uncertainty, support and shame, excitement and fear, power and vulnerability, submission and control, attraction and repulsion, desire and disgust, safety and risk, and life and death. Some months later, instead of a picture, Sessy presented me with a plant. Unbeknown to me, throughout our work together she had patiently tended an avocado stone into a shoot, then a seedling, and now a plant. The stone, with roots submerged in water, still had four sticks embedded in it, like pirate swords piercing its heart. They were keeping the plant from drowning. From the destruction of the shark-infested water came the roots and shoots of physis, the creative growth force of nature: mortido *and* eros, death as well as life.

My relationship with Sessy epitomises for me the message of this book. That client and therapist are both human beings with universal challenges and tensions of existence as well as our own unique history and psychodynamic disturbance. That we all struggle with the shadow of death and destruction, whilst longing to bathe in the light and warmth of creative life, love, and growth. And that therapy is fundamentally about two diverse human beings (who are not that different after all) having an intimate, vulnerable, powerful, creative, and playful conversation about the difficulties, joys, and meaning of life. And the most important message of all? That life – and therapy – is so much more pleasurable when we laugh.

Afterword

The end of the expedition

In the year I have written this book I have experienced a microcosm of life. I have celebrated both my parents' 90th birthdays and have grieved the premature death of my very dear friend. I have tearfully buried my beloved cat in my garden, and, in the same space, have laughed and played with my young great-nephews and nieces. I have held two new great-nieces in my arms, shared the excitement of another niece's first pregnancy, and at the same time supported a much-loved supervisee through recurrent and devastating miscarriages. I have celebrated with loved ones getting married, moving in with their partner, or buying their first home, and cried with those whose family relationships have disintegrated or fractured. I have shared the joy of students and supervisees as they pass their final psychotherapy exams, and been alongside those suffering with the disappointment of deferral. I have endured the painful deterioration through dementia of my mother's memory of her world and of the people she loves, and smiled at my great-nephew bursting with new knowledge and friendships as he started school. I have observed with joy my sons' lives expand as they start new jobs and travel to different continents for the first time, and have been devastated to witness a dear supervisee's too-young life being curtailed following an aggressive incurable cancer diagnosis.

This is life. It is joyful and painful. It is just and unfair. It is kind and cruel. It is invigorating and disturbing. That is just the way it is. For those with psychodynamic disturbance, the difficulties, beauties, and joys of life can sometimes be harder to tolerate or appreciate. But every stage of life brings challenges to us all, whatever our history. We are on our own unique expedition with no idea of the terrain or points of interest we will encounter along the way. The only thing we can be certain about is that this expedition had a start point and will have an ending; yet we do not know how or when it will end, or who will be with us when it does. From conception through to death, things are inflicted upon us that are out of our control, yet we have also ultimately been bequeathed with freedom to choose our subsequent direction. Even then, we are not told the underlying purpose of the mission and have no way of knowing the

DOI: 10.4324/9781003475217-18

outcome of our choices. The responsibility can feel anxiety-provoking. We can feel retrospective guilt for not making the right choices. Life is perplexing, mysterious, precarious, and sometimes torturous. Existence can be a very isolating experience; nobody can help us avoid pain. No expert guide is available to navigate through the terrain because we will inevitably encounter unchartered territory that no soul has lived before. Yet the isolation can be relieved by the company of others. Others who join us in the struggle. Others who have lived, endured, and thrived through similar experiences in life. Others who have gone further in their quest for tolerating the existential tensions of life and can challenge us to do the same. Others who inspire us with their courage in facing death and destruction with equanimity and who have been rewarded with a vibrant passion for living. What a privilege it is to have such a human soul who is willing to accompany us on a leg of our life's pilgrimage. And what a gift it is to be welcomed as that accompanying other.

On a recent expedition to southern Italy, I was exploring the village in which I was staying when I came across a gathered crowd surrounding an empty hearse outside the church on the village square. I noticed passers-by gradually stopping at a respectful distance, and cars and scooters halting in the middle of the street. There was an air of anticipation. I felt like an outsider intruding on a community's ritual, yet it felt rude to leave. And I wanted to stay; I wanted to be part of this community. Then six men carried the coffin from the church. As it emerged, the crowds broke into applause. From the inner circle of mourners, to the villagers enveloping them, to the wider circle of people in surrounding cars and on scooters, from toddler in pushchair to the elderly in wheelchairs, everybody clapped. And I, the alien from outside this community, joined in. As I did so, my foreign status no longer mattered. I was part of a global, universal community that united us. For common to all of us was our humanity, and we were all acknowledging the life and death of a fellow human being, and the grief at their loss that we all knew in our own way. It did not matter that I did not know the person's name, age, gender, cultural heritage, or personal history. I am sure this person lived a life that had moments of both altruism and selfishness, perhaps even magnificence or cruelty. What was significant is that we were all acknowledging that it mattered that they had lived and that they had died, they had existed and were now no longer present in this world. It was right that this small part of the planet stopped for a moment to appreciate that their life had somehow touched the world, and that loved ones and strangers collectively acknowledged the significance of life, death and grief for us all.

I wondered who would clap for me when I died. I wondered whether I would deserve it. And I wondered whether, as my life comes to an end, I will be able to applaud for my own life. I determined there and then to focus on living my life well, to find the most meaning I can in my short existence on earth, to determine to keep growing through the challenges, and to live abundantly, vibrantly, authentically, and with integrity to my own values and beliefs. I hope that, in some way, this book helps you – and the clients you are privileged to accompany – make your own similar but unique choices. Then, perhaps, as our coffins are brought out, it will be appropriate for loved ones, acquaintances, strangers – all fellow humans – to applaud the lives that we have lived.

References

Abram, D. (1997) *The spell of the sensuous: Perception and language in the more-than-human world*. New York: Vintage Books.

Ackerman, D. (1991) *A Natural History of the Senses*. New York: Vintage Books.

Aldridge, B. (2021) 'Core Self, Sense of Self, and Whole Self: The Potential for Harm in Using Personality Disorder Diagnoses', *Transactional Analysis Journal*, *51*(1), pp.49–62. https://doi.org/10.1080/03621537.2020.1853351

Aldridge, B., & Stilman, R. (2024) 'Unmasking Neurodiversity: Revisiting the Relationship Between Core Self and Sense of Self to Examine Common Neurodivergent Script Decisions', *Transactional Analysis Journal*, *54*(1), pp.47–62. https://doi.org/10.1080/03621537.2024.2286576

Aldridge, N. (2024, 19 July–3 November) 'The face of the persecuted' (Natural History Museum's Wildlife Photographer of the Year). Dorset Museum & Art Gallery, Dorchester.

Allen, J. R. (2000) 'Biology and transactional analysis II: A status report on neurodevelopment', *Transactional Analysis Journal*, *30*(4), pp.260–269. https://doi.org/10.1177/036215370003000402

Allen, R. & Allen, B. (1997) 'A New Type of Transactional Analysis and One Version of Script Work with a Constructionist Sensibility', *Transactional Analysis Journal*, *27*(2), pp.89–98.

Anderson, J. (2014) 'Forgiveness – a relational process: Research and reflections', in Loewenthal, D. & Samuels, A. (eds) *Relational psychotherapy, psychoanalysis and counselling: Appraisals and reappraisals*. London & New York: Routledge.

Anderson Stanley, B. (1904/1911) 'What is Success?', in Chapple, J. M. (ed.) *Heart Throbs Volume Two*. New York: Grosset & Dunlap Publishers, pp.1–2.

Angyal, A. (1941) *Foundations for a science of personality*. New York: Commonwealth Fund.

Angyal, A. (1965) *Neurosis and Treatment: A Holistic Theory*. New York: Wiley.

Arendt, H. (1978) *The Life of the Mind. Volume One: Thinking*. Boston: Harcourt.

Arnett, J. J. (2024) *Emerging adulthood: The winding road from the late teens through the twenties* (3rd ed.). Oxford: Oxford University Press. https://doi.org/10.1093/oso/9780197695937.001.0001

Aron, L. (1996) *A meeting of minds: Mutuality in psychoanalysis*. Piedmont, California: Analytic Press, Inc.

Aron, L. (2008) 'The question of technique' (Msg. 13). Message posted to International Association for Relational Psychoanalysis and Psychotherapy colloquium. http://iarpp.net/archive/2008 Dec IC 13.

Atchley, R. C. (1989) 'A continuity theory of normal aging', *Gerontologist*, *29*(2), pp.183–190.

Atchley, R. C. (1997) 'Everyday mysticism: spiritual development of later adulthood', *Journal of Adult Development*, *4*, pp.123–134.

Atlas, G. (2015) 'Touch me, know me: The enigma of erotic longing', *Psychoanalytic Psychology*, *32*, pp.123–139.

Baldwin, J. (1963/2017) *The Fire Next Time*. New York & London: Penguin Random House UK.

Barnes, G. (2004) 'Homosexuality in the First Three Decades of Transactional Analysis: A Study of Theory in the Practice of Transactional Analysis Psychotherapy', *Transactional Analysis Journal*, *34*(2), pp.126–155. DOI:10.1177/036215370403400205

Barr, J. (1987) 'The Therapeutic Relationship Model: Perspectives on the Core of the Healing Process', *Transactional Analysis Journal*, *17*(4), pp.134–140. https://doi.org/10.1177/036215378701700402

Barrow, G. (2014) '"Whatever!" The Wonderful Possibilities of Adolescence', *Transactional Analysis Journal*, *44*(2), pp.167–174. https://doi.org/10.1177/03621537 14543077

Barrow, G. (2020) 'Teaching as Creative Subversion: Education Encounter as an Antidote to Neoliberal Exploitation of the Educational Task', *Transactional Analysis Journal*, *50*(3), pp.179–192.

Barrow, G., & Marshall, H. (2020) 'Ecological transactional analysis: principles for a new movement', *The Transactional Analyst*, *10*(2), pp.5–8.

Barrow, G. & Marshall, H. (2023) 'Revisiting Ecological Transactional Analysis: Emerging Perspectives', *Transactional Analysis Journal*, *53*(1), pp.7–20.

Barsness, R. & Strawn, B. (2018) 'Competency Seven: Courageous speech/disciplined spontaneity', in Barsness, R. (ed.) *Core Competencies of Relational Psychoanalysis A Guide to Practice, Study and Research*. London & New York: Routledge.

Baskerville, V. (2022) A Transcultural and Intersectional Ego State Model of the Self: The Influence of Transcultural and Intersectional Identity on Self and Other. *Transactional Analysis Journal*, *52*(3), pp.228–243. https://doi.org/10.1080/03621537. 2022.2076398

Beauvoir, S. de (1948) *The Ethics of Ambiguity*. New York: Citadel Press Kensington Publishing Corp.

Beauvoir, S. de (1977) *Old Age* (trans. P. O'Brian). Harmondsworth: Penguin.

Becker, E. (1973) *The Denial of Death*. New York: Free Press.

Beekum, S. van (2009) 'Siblings, Aggression, and Sexuality: Adding the Lateral', *Transactional Analysis Journal*, *39*(2), pp.129–135. DOI:10.1177/036215370903 900206

Benjamin, J. (1990) 'An outline of intersubjectivity: The development of recognition', *Psychoanalytic Psychology*, *7* (Suppl.), pp.33–46. https://doi.org/10.1037/h0085258

Berk, L. (2023) *Development Through the Lifespan* (7th ed.). New Jersey: Pearson Education.

Berne, E. (1957) *A Layman's Guide to Psychiatry and Psychoanalysis*. New York: Simon & Schuster.

Berne, E. (1961) *Transactional Analysis in Psychotherapy: A Systematic Individual and Social Psychiatry*. New York: Grove Press.

Berne, E. (1964) *Games people play: The psychology of human relationships*. New York: Grove Press.

Berne, E. (1966) *Principles of Group Treatment*. New York: Oxford University Press.

Berne, E. (1947/1968) *A Layman's Guide to Psychiatry and Psychoanalysis* (3rd ed.). New York: Simon and Schuster. (Original work *The Mind in Action*.)

Berne, E. (1970) *Sex in Human Loving*. New York: Simon and Schuster.

Berne, E. (1971) 'Away from a Theory of the Impact of Interpersonal Interaction on Non-Verbal Participation', *Transactional Analysis Journal, 1*(1), pp.6–13.

Berne, E. (1972/1992) *What do You Say after you Say Hello? The Psychology of Human Destiny*. London: Corgi Books.

Berne, E. (1976) *Beyond Games and Scripts*. New York: Random House.

Berne, E. (1977) *Intuition and ego states*. New York: HarperCollins.

Berry, M. D. (2014) 'Existential psychotherapy and sexual attraction: Meaning and authenticity in the therapeutic encounter', in Luca, M. (ed.) *Sexual Attraction in Therapy, Clinical Perspectives on Moving Beyond the Taboo, A Guide for Training and Practice*. West Sussex: John Wiley & Sons Ltd, pp.38–53.

Biesta, G. J. J. (2014) *The Beautiful Risk of Education*. London: Paradigm.

Binswanger, L. (1942) *Grundformen und Erkenntnis menschlichen Daseins* [*Basic Forms and Knowledge of Human Existence*]. Zürich: Niehans.

Bion, W. R. (1962) *Learning from Experience*. London: Karnac Books.

Blackstone, P. (1993) 'The Dynamic Child: Integration of Second-Order Structure, Object Relations, and Self Psychology', *Transactional Analysis Journal, 23*(4), pp.216–234. https://doi.org/10.1177/036215379302300406

Blake, V. (2017) 'Being With the Emergence of Transgendered Identity', *Transactional Analysis Journal, 47*(4), pp.232–243. DOI:10.1177/0362153717717985

Bollas, C. (1989) *Forces of Destiny: Psychoanalysis and Human Idiom*. London: Free Association Books.

Boss, M. (1977) *I Dreamt Last Night: A New Approach to the Revelations of Dreaming and Its Uses in Psychotherapy* (trans. S. Conway). New York: Gardner Press.

Boss, M. (1979) *Existential Foundations of Medicine and Psychology*. Lanham, Maryland: Jason Aronson, Inc.

Bowater, M. (2008) 'Facing the Fear of Death', *Transactional Analysis Journal, 38*(2), pp.151–154. DOI:10.1177/036215370803800208

Bowie, D. (2022) *Moonage Daydream*. Written, directed and produced by Brett Morgen. HBO Documentary Films.

Bowness, S. (2017) *Barbara Hepworth: The sculptor in the studio*. London: Tate Gallery Publishing.

Brink, D. C. (1987) 'The issues of equality and control in the client- or person-centered approach', *Journal of Humanistic Psychology, 27*(1), pp.27–37. https://doi.org/10.1177/0022167887271003

Browning, R. (1864/2023) '"Rabbi Ben Ezra" in Dramatis Personae, 1864', in Porter, C. & Clarke, H. (eds) *The Poems of Robert Browning*. Independently published.

Buber, M. (1923/1958). *I and Thou* (trans. G. Smith). Edinburgh: T & T Clark.

Buber, M. (1965) *The Knowledge of Man: Selected Essays*. New York: Harper & Row.

Bugental, J. F. T. (1981) *The Search for Authenticity: An Existential-Analytic Approach to Psychotherapy* (Exp. ed.). New York: Irvington.

Buhl, H. M., & Lanz, M. (2007) 'Emerging adulthood in Europe: Common traits and variability across five European countries [Editorial]', *Journal of Adolescent Research, 22*(5), pp.439–443. https://doi.org/10.1177/0743558407306345

Camus, A. (1942/1955) *The myth of Sisyphus* (trans. J. O'Brien). London: Penguin. (Original work *Le Mythe de Sisyphe*.)

Carlsen, M.B. (1988) *Meaning-Making: Therapeutic Processes in Adult Development.* New York: W.W. Norton & Company.

Carlsen, M.B. (1991) *Creative Aging: A Meaning-Making Perspective.* New York: W. W. Norton & Company.

Cazzaniga, M., Jaumotte, F., Li, L., Melina, G., Panton, A.J., Pizzinelli, C., Rockall, E. J., & Tavares, M. M. (2024) Gen-AI: Artificial Intelligence and the Future of Work, *Staff Discussion Notes* 2024, 001. https://doi.org/10.5089/9798400262548.006

Clark, B. (1991) 'Empathic Transactions in the Deconfusion of Child Ego States', *Transactional Analysis Journal, 21*(2), pp.92–98.

Clarkson, P. (1992) *Transactional Analysis Psychotherapy. An Integrated Approach.* London: Tavistock/Routledge.

Clarkson, P. (2003) *The Therapeutic Relationship.* New Jersey & London: Wiley

Clarkson, P. & Fish, S. (1988) 'Rechilding: Creating a New Past in the Present as a Support for the Future', *Transactional Analysis Journal, 18*(1), pp.51–59. https://doi.org/10.1177/036215378801800109

Clarkson, P. & Gilbert, M. (1988) 'Berne's original model of ego states: Some theoretical considerations', *Transactional Analysis Journal, 18*, pp.20–29.

Cohn, H. (1997) *Existential Thought and Therapeutic Practice.* London: Sage.

Colarusso, C. & Nemiroff, R. (1981) *Adult Development: A New Dimension in Psychodynamic Theory and Practice.* New York: Plenum Press.

Collins, N. & Corna, L. (2018) 'General practitioner referral of older patients to Improving Access to Psychological Therapies (IAPT): an exploratory qualitative study', *British Journal of Psychology Bulletin, 42*(3), pp.115 –118. DOI:10.1192/bjb.2018.10

Conway, N. (1978) 'Drivers and Dying', *Transactional Analysis Journal, 8*(4), pp.345–348. DOI:10.1177/036215377800800419

Cook, R. (2012) 'Triumph or disaster?: A relational view of therapeutic mistakes', *Transactional Analysis Journal, 42*(1), pp.34–42.

Cook, R. (2022) 'Connection, Hungers, and Time Structuring: A Relational, Inclusive, and Transpersonal Development of Autonomy', *Transactional Analysis Journal, 52*(4), pp.279–294.

Cook, R. (2023) 'The Development of the Adult Self: An Existential, Relational, and Developmental Approach to Our Human Search for Meaning', *Transactional Analysis Journal, 53*(3), pp.237–255. https://doi.org/10.1080/03621537.2023.2213955

Cooper, J. & Gilbert, M. (2004) 'The role of forgiveness in working with couples', in Ransley, C. & Spy, T. (eds) *Forgiveness and the Healing Process: A Central Therapeutic Concern.* Hove and New York: Brunner-Routledge.

Cooper, M. (2017) *Existential Therapies* (2nd ed.). London: Sage.

Cooper, M. & Adams, M. (2005) 'Death', in van Deurzen, E. & Arnold-Baker, C. (eds) *Existential Perspectives on Human Issues: A Handbook for Therapeutic Practice.* Basingstoke: Palgrave Macmillan.

Corbett, K. (2014) 'The Analyst's Private Space: Spontaneity, Ritual, Psychotherapeutic Action, and Self-Care', *Psychoanalytic Dialogues, 24*(6), pp.637–647. https://doi.org/10.1080/10481885.2014.970964

Cornell, W. F. (1988) 'Life Script Theory: A Critical Review from a Developmental Perspective', *Transactional Analysis Journal, 18*(4), pp.270–282.

Cornell, W.F. (2001) 'There Ain't No Cure without Sex: The Provision of a "Vital" Base', *Transactional Analysis Journal, 31*(4), pp.233–239. DOI:10.1177/036215370 103100405

Cornell, W. F. (2003) 'Babies, brains and bodies: Somatic foundation of the Child', in Sills, C. & Hargaden, H. (eds) *Ego-States*. London: Worth Publishing Ltd.

Cornell, W. F. (2009) 'Why Have Sex?: A Case Study in Character, Perversion, and Free Choice', *Transactional Analysis Journal, 39*(2), pp.136–148. DOI:10.1177/036215370903900207

Cornell, W. F. (2011) 'The impassioned body: Erotic Vitality and Disturbance', Keynote Speech, Humanistic & Integrative Psychotherapy Conference, London, 11 February 2011.

Cornell, W. F. (2013) 'Lost and found: Sibling loss, disconnection, mourning and intimacy', in Frank, A., Clough, P. T., & Seidman, S. (eds) *Intimacies: A New World of Relational Life*. London: Routledge, pp.130–145.

Cornell, W. F. (2014) 'Grief, Mourning, and Meaning', *Transactional Analysis Journal, 44*(4), pp.302–310. DOI:10.1177/0362153714559921

Cornell, W. F. (2015) 'Play at Your Own Risk: Games, Play, and Intimacy', *Transactional Analysis Journal, 45*(2), pp.79–90. https://doi.org/10.1177/0362153715586185

Cornell, W. F. (2020) 'Attribution and alienation: reflections on Claude Steiner's script theory', in Tudor, K. *Claude Steiner, Emotional Activist: The Life and Work of Claude Michel Steiner*. London: Routledge.

Cornell, W. F. & Hargaden, H. (eds) (2019) *The Evolution of a Relational Paradigm in Transactional Analysis: What's the Relationship Got to Do With It?* London: Routledge.

Cornell, W. F. & Landaiche, N. M. III (2006) 'Impasse and Intimacy: Applying Berne's Concept of Script Protocol', *Transactional Analysis Journal, 36* (3), pp.196–213. DOI:10.1177/036215379202200303

Cornell, W. F. & Simerly, T. (2004) 'Letter from the Coeditors', *Transactional Analysis Journal, 34*(2), pp.106–108. DOI:10.1177/036215370403400201

Cowles-Boyd, L. & Boyd, H. S. (1980) 'Play as a time structure', *Transactional Analysis Journal, 10*(1), pp.5–7. https://doi.org/10.1177/036215378001000102

Cox, M. (2001) 'Beyond ego states', *Transactional Analysis UK, 60*, pp.3–8.

Crenshaw, K. (1989) 'Demarginalizing the Intersection of Race and Sex: A Black Feminist Critique of Antidiscrimination Doctrine, Feminist Theory and Antiracist Politics', *University of Chicago Legal Forum, Article 8*.

Crossman, P. (1966) 'Permission and protection', *Transactional Analysis Bulletin, 5*(19), pp.152–154.

Cumming, E. & Henry, W. (1961) *Growing Old: The Process of Disengagement*. New York: Basic Books.

Cymdeithas Eryri Snowdonia Society (2018, 27 July) Cwm Pennant by Eifion Wyn, quoted by Francis, R. in *'Why Lord…'?* blog post.

De La Malla, J. (2024, 19 July–3 November) 'The Dead River' (Natural History Museum's Wildlife Photographer of the Year). Dorset Museum & Art Gallery, Dorchester.

Deaconu, D. (2020) 'The Therapist's Agency as a Subsymbolic Working Tool in the Clinical Encounter: On the Phenomenology of Thinking Martian', *Transactional Analysis Journal, 50*(3), pp.193–206. https://doi.org/10.1080/03621537.2020.1771024

Descartes, R. (1637/1986) *Discourse on Method*. London: Macmillan.

Diehl, M., Coyle, N. & Labouvie-Vief, G. (1996) 'Age and sex differences in strategies of coping and defense across the life span', *Psychology and Aging*, *11*(1), pp.127–139.

Dimen, M. (2024) *Sexuality, Intimacy, Power: Classic Edition*. New York: Routledge.

Du Plock, S. (ed.) (1997) 'Introduction', in *Case studies in Existential Psychotherapy and Counselling*. Chichester: Wiley, pp.1–11.

Eliot, T. S. (1943/2001) 'Little Gidding', in *Four Quartets*. New York: Houghton, Mifflin, Harcourt Publishing Company.

Emin, T. (1998) *My Bed*. Installation view, Tate Britain, London.

English, F. (1971) 'The substitution factor: Rackets and real feelings', *Transactional Analysis Journal*, *1*(4), pp.27–32.

English, F. (1975) 'The Three-Cornered Contract', *Transactional Analysis Journal*, *5*(4), pp.383–384. https://doi.org/10.1177/036215377500500413

English, F (1977) 'What should I do tomorrow? Reconceptualizing transactional analysis', in Barnes, G. (ed.) *Transactional Analysis after Eric Berne*. New York: Harper's College Press, pp.287–327.

English, F. (1988) 'Whither Scripts?', *Transactional Analysis Journal*, *18* (4), pp.294–303.

English, F. (2003) 'How are you? And how am I? Scripts, ego states and inner motivators', in Sills, C. & Hargaden, H. (eds) *Ego states*. Broadway, England: Worth Publishing, pp.55–72.

English, F. (2008) 'Unconscious Drives Reimagined', *Transactional Analysis Journal*, *38*(3), pp.238–246. DOI:10.1177/036215370803800306

Enright, R. D. & Coyle, C. T. (1998) 'Researching the Process Model of Forgiveness within Psychological Interventions', in Worthington, E. L. (ed.) *Dimensions of Forgiveness*. London: Templeton Foundation Press.

Erikson, E. (1950) *Childhood and Society*. London & New York: W. W. Norton & Co.

Erikson, E. (1968) *Identity: Youth and Crisis*. London & New York: W. W. Norton & Co.

Erikson, E. & Erikson, J. (1997) *The Life Cycle Completed*. London and New York: W. W. Norton & Co.

Ermer, A. E., Matera, K. N., & Raymond, S. (2022) 'The reflections on forgiveness framework: A framework to understand older adults' forgiveness development over the life course', *Journal of Adult Development*, *29*(3), pp.255–264. https://doi.org/10.1007/s10804-022-09400-z

Erskine, R. G. (1973) 'Six Stages of Treatment', *Transactional Analysis Journal*, *3*(3), pp.17–18. https://doi.org/10.1177/036215377300300304

Erskine, R.G. (1988) 'Ego Structure, Intrapsychic Function, and Defense Mechanisms: A Commentary on Eric Berne's Original Theoretical Concepts', *Transactional Analysis Journal*, *18*(1), pp.15–19. https://doi.org/10.1177/036215378801800104

Erskine, R.G. (2001) 'Psychological Function, Relational Needs, and Transferential Resolution: Psychotherapy of an Obsession', *Transactional Analysis Journal*, *31*(4), pp.220–226, DOI:10.1177/036215370103100403

Erskine, R. G. (2014) 'What Do You Say Before You Say Good-Bye? The Psychotherapy of Grief', *Transactional Analysis Journal*, *44*(4), pp.279–290. DOI:10.1177/0362153714556622

Erskine, R. G., Clarkson, P., Goulding, R. L., Groder, M. G., & Moiso, C. (1988) 'Ego state theory: Definitions, descriptions, and points of view', *Transactional Analysis Journal*, *18*, pp.6–14.

Erskine, R. G., Moursund, J. P., & Trautmann, R. L. (1999) *Beyond empathy: A therapy of contact-in-relationship*. New York: Brunner/Mazel.

Erskine, R. G. & Zalcman, M. (1979) 'The Racket System: A Model for Racket Analysis', *Transactional Analysis Journal, 9*, pp.51–59.

European Association of Transactional Analysis (2007/2011) 'Ethical code'. https://eatanews.org/wp-content/uploads/2019/04/ethics-code-feb-13th-edit.pdf

Eusden, S. (2021) 'An ethical container for erotic confusion', in Van Rijn, B. & Lukac-Greenwood, J. (eds) *Working with Sexual Attraction in Psychotherapy Practice and Supervision: A Humanistic-Relational Approach*. London: Routledge, pp.195–215.

Eusden, S. (2023) 'High Dare/High Care Compass: A Guide to Transforming Trouble and Ethical Disorientation in Psychotherapy', *Transactional Analysis Journal, 53*(3), pp.207–221.

Fanon, F. (1952/2008) *Black Skin, White Masks* (ed. R. Philcox). New York: Grove Press.

Farber, L. (1967) 'Martin Buber and psychotherapy', in Schilpp, P. A. & Friedman, M. (eds) *The Philosophy of Martin Buber*. LaSalle, IL: Open Court, pp.577–602.

Farber, L. (2000) *The Ways of the Will: Selected essays*. New York: Basic Books.

Foucault, M. (1972) *The Archaeology of Knowledge*. London: Tavistock.

Foucault, M. (1980) *Power/Knowledge: Selected Interviews and other Writings 1972–1977* (trans. C. Gordon, L. Marshall, J. Mepham, & K. Soper). London: Random House Vintage Books.

Fowlie, H., & Sills, C. (eds) (2011) *Relational Transactional Analysis: Principles in Practice*. London: Karnac Books.

Frankl, V. (1946/1969) *Man's Search for Meaning*. London: Hodder & Stoughton.

Freud, S. (1900/1953) *The Interpretation of Dreams* (Standard ed.). London: Hogarth Press.

Freud, S. (1905) *Three Essays on the Theory of Sexuality* (Standard ed.). London: Hogarth Press.

Freud, S. (1937) 'Analysis terminable and interminable', *The International Journal of Psychoanalysis, 18*, pp.373–405.

Freud, S. (1940/1949) *Abriss der psychananalyse* [An outline of psychoanalysis] (trans. J. Strachey). New York: Norton.

Fromm, E. (1955) *The Sane Society*. Austin, Texas: Rinehart & Co..

Fromm, E. (1957) *The Art of Loving*. London: George Allen & Unwin Ltd.

Fromm, E. (1974) *The Anatomy of Human Destructiveness*. London: Jonathan Cape.

Frost, R. (2015) 'The road not taken', in Swank, L. (ed.) *An introduction to American Poetry*. New York: Viking Press, pp.48–49.

Gabbard, G. O. (1994) 'On love and lust in erotic transference', *Journal of the American Psychoanalytic Association, 42*, pp.385–403.

Gabbard, G. O. & Wilkinson, S. M. (1994) *Management of countertransference with borderline patients*. Washington: American Psychiatric Association.

Gadamer, H. (2004) *Truth and Method*. London: Continuum.

Gans, S. (2015) 'Awakening to love: R.D. Laing's phenomenological therapy', in Thompson, M. G. (ed.) *The Legacy of R.D. Laing: An Appraisal of his Contemporary Relevance*. Hove, England: Routledge.

Garcia, F. (2012) 'Healing Good-Byes and Healthy Hellos: Learning and Growing from Painful Endings and Transitions', *Transactional Analysis Journal, 42*(1), pp.53–61. DOI: 10.1177/036215371204200107

Gogh, V. van (1883) 'Letter 301', in Jansen, L., Luijten, H. & Bakker, N. (eds) *Vincent van Gogh: The Letters. The complete, illustrated and annotated edition* (English ed.). London: Thames and Hudson, 2009.

Gollnick, J. (2008) *Religion and Spirituality in the Life Cycle*. New York: Peter Lang.

Goulding, R. & Goulding, M. (1978) *The Power is in the Patient: A TA/Gestalt Approach to Psychotherapy*. San Francisco: TA Press.

Goulding, M. & Goulding, R. (1979) *Changing Lives Through Redecision Therapy*. Hove, UK: Brunner/Mazel.

Graham, D. W. (2023) 'Heraclitus (n.d.)', in Zalta, E. N. (ed.) (2023) *Stanford Encyclopedia of Philosophy*. https://plato.stanford.edu/entries/heraclitus/

Gubi, P. M. (2015) *Spiritual Accompaniment and Counselling: Journeying with Psyche and Soul*. London and Philadelphia: Jessica Kingsley Publishers.

Hargaden, H. (2001) 'There Ain't No Cure for Love: The Psychotherapy of an Erotic Transference', *Transactional Analysis Journal, 31*(4), pp.213–219. DOI:10.1177/036215370103100402

Hargaden, H. (2011) 'The erotic relational matrix revisited', in Fowlie, H. & Sills, C. (eds) *Relational Transactional Analysis: Principles in Practice*. London: Karnac Books, pp.233–248.

Hargaden, H. & Sills, S. (2001) 'Deconfusion of the Child Ego State: A Relational Perspective', *Transactional Analysis Journal, 31*(1), pp.55–70.

Hargaden, H., & Sills, C. (2002) *Transactional Analysis: A Relational Perspective*. Hove, UK: Brunner-Routledge.

Hargreaves, R. (1976) *Mr Mean*. US: Price Stern Sloan.

Havighurst, R.J. (1972) *Developmental tasks and education*. Philadelphia: McKay.

Heath, L. (2014) 'Keeping Our Balance: The profound challenge of loss', *Transactional Analysis Journal, 44*(4), pp.291–301. DOI:10.1177/0362153714559922

Heathcote, A. (2016) 'Eric Berne and Loss', *Transactional Analysis Journal, 46*(3), pp.232–243. DOI:10.1177/0362153716648979

Hegel, G. W. F. (1807/2016) *The Phenomenology of Spirit (The Phenomenology of Mind)* (trans J. B. Baillie). North Charleston, South Carolina: CreateSpace Independent Publishing. (Original work *Phänomenologie des Geistes*.)

Heidegger, M. (1927/2010) *Being and Time* (trans. Joan Stambaugh). New York: State University of New York Press.

Heidegger, M. (1935/1987) *An Introduction to Metaphysics* (trans. R. Manheim). New Haven, CT: Yale University Press.

Heiller, B. & Sills, C. (2010) 'Lifescripts: an existential perspective', in Erskine, R. (ed.) *Life Scripts: A Transactional Analysis of Unconscious Relational Patterns*. London: Karnac Books.

Hemingway, E. (1929) *A Farewell to Arms*. London: Cape.

Hemlin, T. (2012) 'Relational Impasse: Understanding Couple Dynamics Using Impasse Theory Interpersonally', *Transactional Analysis Journal, 42*(2), pp.118–125.

Hepworth, B. (2012) *Barbara Hepworth: A Pictorial Autobiography*. London: Tate Publishing.

Hicklin, A. (2016, 11 January) 'Interview with David Bowie for Gear Magazine, 1999', in *David Bowie, An Obituary*. New York: Bob Guccione, Jr.

Hine, J. (1997) 'Mind Structure and Ego States', *Transactional Analysis Journal, 27*(4), pp.278–289.

Hoffman, P. (1993) 'Death, time, history: Division II of *Being and Time*', in Guignon, C. B. (ed.) *The Cambridge Companion to Heidegger*. Cambridge: Cambridge University Press.

Holtby, M. (1979) 'Interlocking Racket Systems', *Transactional Analysis Journal*, 9(2), pp.131–135.

Holy Bible, *New Living Translation* (1996) Il, US: Tyndale House Publishers.

Hoogendijk, A. (1988) *Spreekuur bij een filosoof* [Philosophical Counselling]. Utrecht: Veers.

Hughes, T. P. (1991). Acceptance. *Science, Technology, & Human Values, 16*(3), pp.387–389. https://doi.org/10.1177/016224399101600308

Hunt, J. & Sills, C. (2021) 'The supervisory dimension', in Van Rijn, B. & Lukac-Greenwood, J. (eds) *Working with Sexual Attraction in Psychotherapy Practice and Supervision: A Humanistic-Relational Approach*. London: Routledge, pp.99–114.

Husserl, E. (1931/2012) *Ideas: General introduction to pure phenomenology*, vol. 1. (trans. D. Moran). London: Routledge.

Ihde, D. (1986) *Experimental Phenomenology: An introduction*. Albany: State University of New York.

International Transactional Analysis Association (2014) 'Code of ethical conduct'. https://itaaworld.com/wp-content/uploads/2023/05/12-5-14-Revised-Ethics_0.pdf

Jaques, E. (1965) 'Death and the mid-life crisis', *The International Journal of Psychoanalysis, 46*(4), pp.502–514.

Isaacowitz, D. M., Vicaria, I. M., & Murry, M. W. E. (2016) 'A lifespan developmental perspective on interpersonal accuracy', in J. A. Hall, M. S. Mast, & T. V. West (eds) *The Social Psychology of Perceiving Others Accurately*. Cambridge: Cambridge University Press, pp.206–229. https://doi.org/10.1017/CBO9781316181959.010

Jaspers, K. (1925/1960) *Psychologie der Weltanschauungen*. Berlin: Springer.

Jenkins, P. (2006) 'Contracts, Ethics and the Law', in Sills, C. (ed.) *Contracts in Counselling & Psychotherapy*. London: Sage.

Johnson, S. (2004) 'From Cultural Scripting to Autonomy: Influences on Lesbian Identity', *Transactional Analysis Journal*, 34(2), pp.170–179. DOI:10.1177/03621 5370403400207

Johnson, S. (2017) 'The Trouble With Gender', *Transactional Analysis Journal*, 47:4, 308–320. DOI:10.1177/0362153717725533

Jung, C. G. (1912/2023) *The Psychology of the Unconsciou*. (trans. B. Hinkle). London: Valde Books.

Jung, C. G. (1963) *Memories, Dreams, Reflections*. London: Collins Fountain Books.

Jung, C. G. (1931/1970) *Collected Works of C.G. Jung, Volume 8: The Structure and Dynamics of the Psyche*, Bollingen Series (ed. and trans. G. Adler & R. F. C. Hull). Princeton, New Jersey: Princeton University Press. (Original work *The Stages of Life*.)

Karpman, S. B. (2010) 'Intimacy analysis today: The intimacy scale and the personality pinwheel', *Transactional Analysis Journal*, 40(3–4), pp.224–242.

Kastenbaum, R. (ed.) (1964) *New Thoughts on Old Age*. New York: Springer.

Kaye, J. (1995) 'Postfoundationalism and the language of psychotherapy research', in J. Siegfried (ed.) *Therapeutic and Everyday Discourse as Behavior Change: Towards a Micro-Analysis in Psychotherapy Process Research*. New York: Ablex Publishing.

Kegan, R. (1982) *The Evolving Self: Problem and Process in Human Development*. Cambridge, Massachusetts, London: Harvard University Press.

Kegan, R. & Lahey, L. (2009) *Immunity to Change: How to Overcome It and Unlock the Potential in Yourself and Your Organization*. Boston: Harvard Business Press.

Kellett, P. (2004) 'Queer Constructions: The Making of Gay Men and the Role of the Homoerotic in Therapy', *Transactional Analysis Journal*, *34*(2), pp.180–190. DOI:10.1177/036215370403400208

Kierkegaard, S. (1843/1987) *Either/Or. Part 1*. (ed. and trans. H. V. Hong & E. H. Hong). Princeton, NJ: Princeton University Press.

Kierkegaard, S. (1844/1980) *The Concept of Anxiety* (trans. R. Thomte). Princeton, NJ: Princeton University Press.

King, S. (1983) *Christine*. New York: Signet.

Klein, M. (1948) 'A contribution to the theory of anxiety and guilt', *The International Journal of Psychoanalysis*, *29*, pp.114–123.

Kohut, H. (1971) *The Analysis of the Self: A Systematic Approach to the Psychoanalytic Treatment of Narcissistic Personality Disorder*. New York: International Universities Press.

Krook, J. (2021, 26 April) 'The Art of Paul Cezanne', in New Intrigue: Literature, Philosophy, Technology blog.

Kuchuck, S. (2014) *Clinical Implications of the Psychoanalyst's Life Experience: When the Personal Becomes Professional*. New York: Routledge.

Kupfer, D. & Haimowitz, M. (1971) 'Therapeutic Interventions Part I. Rubberbands Now', *Transactional Analysis Journal*, *1*(2), pp.10–16. https://doi.org/10.1177/036215377100100205

Kunnen, E. S., Sappa, V., Geert, P. L. C., & Bonica, L. (2008) 'The shapes of commitment development in emerging adulthood', *Journal of Adult Development*, 15, pp.113–131.

Labouvie-Vief, G. (2006) 'Emerging Structures of Adult Thought', in Arnett, J. J. & Tanner, J. L. (eds) *Emerging adults in America: Coming of age in the 21st century*. Washington: American Psychological Association, pp.59–84. https://doi.org/10.1037/11381-003

Laing, R. D. (1960) *The Divided Self*. London: Penguin.

Laing, R. D. & Esterson, A. (1964) *Sanity, Madness and the Family*. London: Tavistock Publications.

Lankford, V. (1980) 'Termination: How to Enrich the Process', *Transactional Analysis Journal*, *10*(2), pp.175–177. DOI:10.1177/036215378001000224

Larner, G. (1999) 'Derrida and the deconstruction of power as context and topic in therapy', in Parker, I. (ed.) *Deconstructing Psychotherapy*. London & California: SAGE Publications Ltd, pp.39–53. https://doi.org/10.4135/9781446217962

Lee, A. (2006) 'Process contracts', in Sills, C. (ed.) *Contracts in Counselling & Psychotherapy*. London: Sage.

Leigh, E. (2011) 'The censorship process: from distillation to essence – a relational methodology', in Fowlie, H. & Sills, C. (eds) *Relational Transactional Analysis: Principles in Practice*. London: Karnac Books.

Lemish, D. & Muhlbauer, V. (2012) '"Can't Have it All": Representations of Older Women in Popular Culture', *Women & Therapy*, *35*(3–4), pp.165–180. https://doi.org/10.1080/02703149.2012.684541

Levin, P. (2003) 'What Does it Mean to Be an Adult?', *Transactional Analysis Journal*, *33*(1), pp.76–78. https://doi.org/10.1177/036215370303300111

Levin, P. (2015) 'Ego States and Emotional Development in Adolescence', *Transactional Analysis Journal*, *45*(3), pp.228–237. https://doi.org/10.1177/0362153715599990

Levin-Landheer, P. (1982) 'The Cycle of Development', *Transactional Analysis Journal*, *12*(2), pp.129–139. https://doi.org/10.1177/036215378201200207

Levinson, D. J. (1978) *Seasons of a Man's Life*. New York: Random House.

Levinson, D. J. (1986) 'A conception of adult development', *American Psychologist*, *41*(1), pp.3–13. https://doi.org/10.1037/0003-066X.41.1.3

Levinson, D. J. (1996) *Seasons of a Woman's Life*. New York: Alfred A. Knopf.

Levitt, M. J. & Cici-Gokaltun, A. (2011) 'Close relationships across the life span', in Fingerman, K. L., Berg, C. A., Smith, J., & Antonucci, T. C. (eds) *Handbook of Life-Span Development*. New York: Springer Publishing Company, pp.457–486.

Lewis, C. S. (1960/2002) *The Four Loves*. London: HarperCollins Publishers.

Lewis, C. S. (2000) *Collected letters Vol.1: Family letters 1905–1931* (ed. Walter Hooper). London: HarperCollins Publishers.

Lewis, M. A., Granato, H., Blayney, J. A., Lostutter, T. W., & Kilmer, J. R. (2012) 'Predictors of hooking up sexual behaviors and emotional reactions among U.S. college students', *Archives of Sexual Behavior*, *41*, pp.1219–1229.

Little, R. (2006) 'Ego State Relational Units and Resistance to Change', *Transactional Analysis Journal*, *36*(1), pp.7–19.

Little, R. (2011) 'Impasse Clarification within the Transference-Countertransference Matrix', *Transactional Analysis Journal*, *41*(1), pp.23–38. https://doi.org/10.1177/036215371104100106

Little, R. (2018) 'The Management of Erotic/Sexual Countertransference Reactions: An Exploration of the Difficulties and Opportunities Involved', *Transactional Analysis Journal*, *48*(3), pp.224–241. DOI:10.1080/03621537.2018.1471290

Lomas, P. (1981) *The Case for a Personal Psychotherapy*. Oxford: Oxford University Press.

Loomis, M. (1982) 'Contracting for Change', *Transactional Analysis Journal*, *12*(1), pp.51–55. https://doi.org/10.1177/036215378201200107

Madison, G.B. (1981) *Phenomenology of Merleau-Ponty: Search for the Limits of Consciousness*. Athens, Ohio: Ohio University Press.

Mann, D. (1997) *Psychotherapy: An Erotic Relationship – Transference and Countertransference Passions*. London: Routledge.

Mannix, K. (2022) *With the End in Mind: How to Live and Die Well*. London and Dublin: William Collins.

Marcel, G. (1964) *Creative Fidelity* (trans. R. Rosthal). New York: Farrar, Strauss and Company.

Margulies, A. (1989) *The Empathic Imagination*. New York: W. W. Norton.

Maroda, K. J. (1999) *Seduction, Surrender, and Transformation: Emotional Engagement in the Analytic Process*. Piedmont, California: Analytic Press.

Marshall, A. & Milton, M. (2014) 'Therapists' disclosures and their sexual feelings to their clients: The importance of honesty – An interpretative phenomenological approach', in Luca, M. (ed.) *Sexual Attraction in Therapy, Clinical Perspectives on Moving Beyond the Taboo, A Guide for Training and Practice*. West Sussex: John Wiley & Sons Ltd, pp.209–226.

Maslow, A. (1962) *Toward a Psychology of Being*. New York: D. Van Nostrand. https://doi.org/10.1037/10793-000

Massey, R. F. (2007) 'Re-examining social psychiatry as a foundational framework for transactional analysis: Considering a social-psychological perspective', *Transactional Analysis Journal*, *37*, pp.51–79.

May, R. (1961) 'Existential psychiatry an evaluation', *Journal of Religion and Health*, 1, pp.31–40. https://doi.org/10.1007/BF01532010

May, R. (1969) *Love and Will*. New York and London: W. W. Norton & Co.

May, R. (1977) *The meaning of anxiety* (Rev. ed.). New York and London: W. W. Norton & Co.

May, R., Angel, E., & Ellenbrger, H. F. (eds) (1958). *Existence*. New York: Basic Books.

McFadden, S. H. (1999) 'Religion, personality and aging: a life span perspective', *Journal of Personality* 67(6), pp.1081–1104.

McLean, B. (2017) 'Oedipal Wrecks, the AIDS Crisis, and the Diagnosis of Gender Incongruence', *Transactional Analysis Journal*, *47*(4), pp.251–263. DOI:10.1177/0362153717720190

McQuaid, C. (2021) *Understanding Bereaved Parents and Siblings: A Handbook for Professionals, Families and Friends*. Oxon: Routledge.

Mearns, D. & Cooper, M. (2005) *Working at Relational Depth in Counselling and Psychotherapy*. London: Sage.

Mellor, K. (1980) 'Impasses: A Developmental and Structural Understanding', *Transactional Analysis Journal*, *10*(3), pp.213–220.

Menon, U. (2015) 'Midlife narratives across cultures: Decline or pinnacle?', in Jensen, L. A. (ed.) *The Oxford Handbook of Human Development and Culture: An Interdisciplinary Perspective*. Oxford: Oxford University Press, pp.637–652.

Merleau-Ponty, M. (1945/1962) *Phenomenology of Perception*. London: Routledge.

Merriam-Webster.com (2023) 'Encounter'. https://www.merriam-webster.com/dictionary/encounter

Metropolitan Museum of Art (2024) 'The Houses of Parliament'. https://www.metmuseum.org/art/collection/search/437128

Miller, D. A. (1981) 'The "sandwich" generation: adult children of the aging', *Social Work*, 26(5), pp.419–423.

Milton, M. (2014), Introduction – Sexuality: Debates and controversies', in Milton, M. (ed.) *Sexuality: Existential Perspectives*. Monmouth: PCCS Books Ltd, pp.1–20.

Minikin, K. (2008) 'Treatment planning', *ITA News*, *37*(2), pp.13–14.

Minikin, K. (2018) 'Radical relational psychiatry: Toward a democracy of mind and people', *Transactional Analysis Journal*, *48*(2), pp.111–125.

Minikin, K. (2021) 'Treatment Planning: Pathway to Cure?', *Transactional Analysis Journal*, *51*(3), pp.254–266.

Minikin, K. (2023) *Radical-Relational Perspectives in Transactional Analysis Psychotherapy: Oppression, Alienation, Reclamation*. Oxon and New York: Routledge.

Mitchell, S. A. (1988) *Relational Concepts in Psychoanalysis: An Integration*. Massachusetts & London: Harvard University Press.

Moiso, C. (1985) 'Ego States and Transference', *Transactional Analysis Journal*, *15*(3), pp.194–201. https://doi.org/10.1177/036215378501500302

Mothersole, G. (1996) 'Existential Realities and No-Suicide Contracts', *Transactional Analysis Journal*, *26*(2), pp.151–159. DOI:10.1177/036215379602600206

Mothersole, G. (2006) 'Contracts and harmful behaviour', in Sills, C. (ed.) *Contracts in Counselling & Psychotherapy*. London: Sage.

Mowzat, H. (2005) 'Ageing, spirituality and health', *Scottish Journal of Healthcare Chaplaincy*, *8*(1), pp.7–12.

Mullan, B. (1997) 'Interview with M. Semyon', in Mullan, B. (ed.) *R.D. Laing: Creative Destroyer*. London & California: Sage Publications Ltd.

Mullen, J. D. (1995) *Kierkegaard's Philosophy: Self Deception and Cowardice in the Present Age*. Maryland: University Press of America.

Nelson, T. D. (2011) 'Ageism: the strange case of prejudice against the older you', in Wiener, R. L. & Willbourne, S. L. (eds) *Disability and Aging Discrimination*. New York: Springer.

Neugarten, B. L. (1968) *Middle Age and Aging: A Reader in Social Psychology*. Chicago, IL: University of Chicago Press.

Neugarten, B. L. (1975) 'The future and the young-old', *The Gerontologist*, *15*(1, Pt 2), pp.4–9.

Neugarten, B. L. (1979) 'Time, age, and the life cycle', *The American Journal of Psychiatry*, *136*(7), pp.887–894.

New King James Version Holy Bible (1982) London: HarperCollins.

Newton, T. (2006) 'Script, Psychological Life Plans, and the Learning Cycle', *Transactional Analysis Journal*, *36*(3), pp.186–195. https://doi.org/10.1177/036215370603600303

Nietzsche, F. (1883/1969) *Thus Spake Zarathustra* (trans. R. J. Hollingdale). Harmondsworth: Penguin Books.

Nietzsche, F. (1886/1989) *Beyond good and evil* (trans. H. Zimmern). New York: Prometheus,

Northoff, G. (2018) *The Spontaneous Brain: From the Mind-Body to the World-Brain Problem*. Cambridge, Massachusetts, MIT Press.

Novak, E. T. (2015) 'Are games, enactments, and reenactments similar? No, yes, it depends', *Transactional Analysis Journal*, *45*(2), pp.117–127.

Novak, E. T. (2016) 'When Transgressing Standard Therapeutic Frames Leads to Progressive Change, Not Ethical Violations: Secret Garden Work', *Transactional Analysis Journal*, *46*(4), pp.288–298. https://doi.org/10.1177/0362153716662267

Novalis (2007) *Notes for a Romantic Encyclopaedia: Das Allgemeine Brouillon* (ed. and trans. David Wood). Albany: State University of New York Press.

Novellino, M. (2008) 'A Transactional Psychoanalysis of Frodo: The Conflict of the Male Adolescent in Becoming a Man', *Transactional Analysis Journal*, *38*(3), pp.233–237. https://doi.org/10.1177/036215370803800305

Nuttall, J. (2006) 'The Existential Phenomenology of Transactional Analysis', *Transactional Analysis Journal*, *36*(3), pp.214–227.

Oates, S. & Kuchuck, S. (2016) 'Privacy, Hiding, Silencing, and Self-Revelation: A Conversation Between Steven Kuchuck and Steff Oates', *Transactional Analysis Journal*, *46*(4), pp.355–361. https://doi.org/10.1177/0362153716665586

Ohshima, A. (2024, 19 July–3 November) 'Forest Rodeo' (Natural History Museum's Wildlife Photographer of the Year). Dorset Museum & Art Gallery.

Orbach, A. (1999) *Life, Psychotherapy and Death: The End of Our Exploring*. London: Jessica Kingsley.

O'Shea, L. (2000) 'Sexuality: Old Struggles and New Challenges', *Gestalt Review*, *4*(8). 10.5325/gestaltreview.4.1.0008

Pearce, R. (2011) 'Escaping into the other: an existential view of sex and sexuality', *Existential Analysis*, *22*(2), p.229.

Peavey, F. (1997) 'Strategic Questioning Manual'. Gestalt Therapy International. https://www.gti.today/Resources/strategic_questioning.pdf

Piaget, J. (1971). 'The theory of stages in cognitive development', in Green, D. R., Ford, M. P. & G. B. Flamer, G. B. *Measurement and Piaget*. New York: McGraw-Hill.

Plath, S. (1967) *The Bell Jar*. London: Faber & Faber.

Plato (1993) *The Symposium and The Phaedrus: Plato's Erotic Dialogues*. Albany: State University of New York Press.

Pope, K. S. & Bouhoutsos, J. C. (1986) *Sexual intimacy between therapists and patients*. New York and London: Praeger Publishers.

Prensky, M. (2001) 'Digital Natives, Digital Immigrants, Part 1', *On The Horizon*, 9, pp.3–6. http://dx.doi.org/10.1108/10748120110424816

Proctor, G. (2017) *The Dynamics Of Power In Counselling And Psychotherapy* (2nd ed.). Monmouth: PCCS Books.

Quinodoz, D. (2010) *Growing Old: A journey Of Self-Discovery* (trans. D. Alcorn). London & New York: Routledge.

Radhakrishnan, S. (1989) *Indian Philosophy*. London: Unisin Hyman.

Rank, O. (1945) *Will Therapy and Truth and Reality*. New York: Alfred A. Knopf.

Ransley, C. & Spy, T. (eds) (2004) *Forgiveness and the Healing Process: A Central Therapeutic Concern*. Hove, UK: Brunner-Routledge.

Read, J. (1961) *Barbara Hepworth*. British Broadcasting Corporation (BBC).

Ricoeur, P. (2007) *Vivant jusqu' à la mort* [Living Until Death Comes]. Paris: Le Seuil.

Rogers, C. R. (1959) 'A theory of therapy, personality, and interpersonal relationships as developed in the client-centered framework', in S. Koch (ed.) *Psychology: A study of a Science, Formulations of the Person and the Social Context*. New York: McGraw-Hill, Vol. 3, pp.184–256.

Rogers, C. R. (1963) 'The concept of the fully functioning person', *Psychotherapy*, 1(1), pp.17–26.

Rogers, C. (1990) 'This is me', in Kirschenbaum, H. & Henderson, V. L. (eds) *The Carl Rogers Reader*. London: Constable, pp.6–28.

Rosario, V. A. (2017) 'Historical and Clinical Experiences Across the Gender Spectrum', *Transactional Analysis Journal*, 47(4), pp.244–250. DOI:10.1177/0362153717719031

Rowland, R. & Cornell, W. F. (2021) 'Gender Identity, Queer Theory, and Working With the Sociopolitical in Counseling and Psychotherapy: Why There Is No Such Thing As Neutral', *Transactional Analysis Journal*, 51(1), pp.19–34. DOI:10.1080/03 621537.2020.1853347

Sartre, J.-P. (1943/1956) *Being and Nothingness*. New York: Philosophical Library.

Sartre, J-P. (1946/2007. *Existentialism Is a Humanism*. New Haven: Yale University Press.

Sartre, J-P. (1957) 'The Humanism of Existentialism', in Guignon, C. G. & Pereboom, D. *Existentialism Basic Writings* (trans. B. Frechtman). Indianapolis, IA: Hackett, pp.290–308.

Satir, V. (1964) *Conjoint Family Therapy*. Palo Alto, CA: Science and Behavior Books.

Satir, V. (1988) *The New Peoplemaking*. Palo Alto, CA: Science & Behavior Books.

Schiff, J. L. (with Schiff, A. W., Mellor, K., Schiff, E., Schiff, S., Richman, D., Fishman, J., Wolz, L., Fishman, C., & Momb, D.) (1975) *Cathexis Reader: Transactional Analysis Treatment of Psychosis*. New York: Harper & Row.

Schneider, K. (ed.) (2008) *Existential-Integrative Psychotherapy: Guideposts to the Core of Practice*. New York: Routledge.

Schneider, K. (2023) *Life Enhancing Anxiety: Key to a Sane World*. Colorado: University Professors Press.

Schore, A. N. (2019) *Right Brain Psychotherapy*. London & New York: W.W. Norton.

Schreiber, G. (1936) *Portraits and Self-Portraits*. Boston: Houghton Mifflin Company.

Shah, A., Kosinski, M., Stillwell, D., Seligman, M. E., & Ungar, L.H. (2013) 'Personality, gender, and age in the language of social media: the open-vocabulary approach', *PLoS One, 25*(8), p.9.

Scott, A. J. & Gratton, L. (2021) *The New Long Life: A Framework for Flourishing in a Changing World*. London: Bloomsbury Publishing.

Sedgwick, J. (2021) *Contextual Transactional Analysis: The Inseparability of Self and World*. Oxon, and New York: Routledge.

Seligman, M. (2011) *Flourish: A Visionary New Understanding of Happiness and Well-Being*. New York: Free Press.

Shadbolt, C. (2004) 'Homophobia and Gay Affirmative Transactional Analysis', *Transactional Analysis Journal, 34*(2), pp.113–125. DOI:10.1177/036215370403400204

Shadbolt, C. (2009) 'Sexuality and Shame', *Transactional Analysis Journal, 39*(2), pp.163–172. DOI:10.1177/036215370903900210

Shadbolt, C. (2012) 'The place of failure and rupture in psychotherapy', *Transactional Analysis Journal, 42*(1), pp.5–16.

Shadbolt, C. (2017) 'Dancing in a Different Country', *Transactional Analysis Journal, 47*(4), pp.264–275. DOI:10.1177/0362153717719030

Shadbolt, C. (2021) 'The disturbance and comfort of forbidden conversations (sexuality and erotic forces in relational psychotherapy supervision)', in Van Rijn, B. & Lukac-Greenwood, J. (eds) *Working with Sexual Attraction in Psychotherapy Practice and Supervision: A Humanistic-Relational Approach*. London: Routledge, pp.115–133.

Sheehy, G. (2006) *Passages: Predictable Crises of Adult Life*. New York: Ballantine Books.

Shivanath, S. & Hiremath, M. (2003) 'The psychodynamics of race and culture: An analysis of cultural scripting and ego state transference', in Sills, C. & Hargaden, H. (eds) *Ego States* (Key Concepts in Transactional Analysis: Contemporary Views). London: Worth, pp.169–184..

Siegel, D. (2020) *The Developing Mind: How Relationships and the Brain Interact to Shape Who We Are*. New York: Guilford Press.

Sills, C. (2001) 'The Man with No Name: A Response to Hargaden and Erskine', *Transactional Analysis Journal, 31*(4), pp.227–232. DOI:10.1177/036215370103100404

Sills, C. (2006) 'Contracts and Contract-Making', in Sills, C. (ed.) *Contracts in Counselling & Psychotherapy*. London: Sage.

Sills, C., & Stuthridge, J. (2016) 'Psychological games and intersubjective processes', in Erskine, R. G. (ed.) *Transactional Analysis in Contemporary Psychotherapy*. London: Routledge, pp.185–208..

Simpson, S. W. (2023) 'Introduction', in Simpson, S. W., Racho, M., Robbins, B. D., & Hoffman, L. (Eds) *Eros & Psyche: Existential Perspectives on Sexuality, Volume 1 Philosophical & Theoretical Perspectives*. Colorado: University Professors Press.

Smith-Pickard, P. (2014) 'Merleau-Ponty and Existential Sexuality', in Milton, M. (ed.) *Sexuality: Existential Perspectives*. Monmouth: PCCS Books.

Snyder, J. S. & Cameron, H. A. (2012) 'Could adult hippocampal neurogenesis be relevant for human behavior?', *Behavioural Brain Research, 227*, pp.384–390.

Spinelli, E. (1994) *Demystifying therapy*. London: Constable Publishers.

Spinelli, E. (2001) *The mirror and the Hammer: Challenges to Therapeutic Orthodoxy*. London: Continuum.

Spinelli, E. (2005) *The Interpreted World: An Introduction to Phenomenological Psychology*. London: Sage.

Spinelli, E. (2014) 'Being Sexual: Reconfiguring human sexuality', in Milton, M. (ed.) *Sexuality: Existential Perspectives*. Monmouth: PCCS Books, pp.21–61.

Spinelli, E. (2015) *Practising Existential Therapy* (2nd ed.). London: Sage.

Stace, W. T. (1920) *A Critical History of Greek Philosophy*. London: Macmillan & Co. Ltd.

Stark, M. (2000) *Modes of Therapeutic Action*. NJ Northvale: Jason Aronson.

Steiner, C. (1966) 'Script and counterscript', *Transactional Analysis Bulletin*, *5*(18), pp.133–135.

Steiner, C. (1968) 'Transactional analysis as a treatment philosophy', *Transactional Analysis Bulletin*, 7(27), pp.61–64.

Steiner, C. (1974) *Scripts People Live: Transactional Analysis of Life Scripts*. New York: Grove Press.

Steiner, C. (1979) *Healing Alcoholism*. London: Grove Press.

Steiner, C. (1986) *When a Man loves a Woman: Sexual and Emotional Literacy for the Modern Man*. London: Grove Press.

Steiner, C. M. (1987) 'The Seven Sources of Power: An Alternative to Authority', *Transactional Analysis Journal*, *17*(3), pp.102–104. https://doi.org/10.1177/0362153 78701700309

Steiner, C., Wyckoff, H., D. Goldstine, Lariviere, P., Schwebel, R., & Marcus, J. (1969/1975) *Readings in Radical Psychiatry*. New York: Grove Press.

Stern, D. N. (1985) *The Interpersonal World of the Infant: A View from Psychoanalysis and Developmental Psychology*. New York: Basic Books.

Stern, D. (1998) *The Interpersonal World of the Infant: A View from Psychoanalysis and Developmental Psychology*. London: Karnac Books.

Stern, D. (2004a) *The Present Moment in Psychotherapy and Everyday Life*. New York: W.W. Norton & Co.

Stern, D. B. (2004b) 'The Eye Sees Itself: Dissociation, Enactment, and the Achievement of Conflict', *Contemporary Psychoanalysis*, *40*(2), pp.197–237. https://doi.org/10.1080/ 00107530.2004.10745828

Stewart, I. (1996) 'Book Review: Good Grief Rituals: Tools for Healing', *Transactional Analysis Journal*, *26*(3), pp.270–271. DOI:10.1177/036215379602600316

Stewart, I. (2007) *Transactional Analysis Counselling in Action*. London: Sage.

Summers, G. & Tudor, K. (2000) 'Cocreative Transactional Analysis', *Transactional Analysis Journal*, 30(1), pp.23–40.

Suriyaprakash, C. & Geetha, R. S. (2014) 'Embracing Eternity', *Transactional Analysis Journal*, 44(4), pp.334–346. DOI:10.1177/0362153714560336

Taine, H. (1864) *Voyage en Italie. Tome I: Naples et Rome; Tome II: Florence et Venice*. Paris: Librairie de l. Hachette et Cie.

Thomas, D. (1937/2003) 'Do not go gentle into that good night', in *The Poems of Dylan Thomas* (ed. John Goodby). New York: New Directions Publishers.

Tillich, P. (1952) *The Courage To Be*. Glasgow: Penguin Classics.

Tillich, P. (1954) *Love, Power, and Justice*. New York: Oxford University Press.

Tornstam, L. (2005) *Gerotranscendence: A Developmental Theory of Positive Aging*. New York: Springer Publishing Company.

Tournier, P. (1972) *Learn to Grow Old*. New York: Harper & Row.

Tudor, K. (1995) 'What Do You Say about Saying Good-Bye?: Ending Psychotherapy', *Transactional Analysis Journal*, 25(3), pp.228–233. DOI:10.1177/036215379502500307

Tudor, K. (2003) 'The neopsyche: The integrating adult ego state', in Sills, C. & Hargaden, H. (eds) *Ego States. Key Concepts in Transactional Analysis: Contemporary Views*. London: Worth, pp.201–231.

Tudor, K. (2006) 'Contracts, complexity and challenge', in Sills, C. (ed.) Contracts in Counselling and Psychotherapy (2nd ed.). London: Sage, pp.119–136.

Tudor, K. (2010) 'The State of the Ego: Then and Now', *Transactional Analysis Journal*, 40(3–4), pp.261–277.

Tudor, K. (2011) 'Understanding empathy', *Transactional Analysis Journal*, 41(1), pp.39–57.

Tudor, K., & Summers, G. (2014) *Co-creative Transactional Analysis: Papers, Responses, Dialogues and Developments*. London: Karnac Books.

Tudor, K. & Widdowson, M. (2001) 'Integrating Views of TA Brief Therapy', in K. Tudor (ed.) *Transactional Analysis Approaches to Brief Therapy*. London: Sage.

Vaillant, G. E. (2002) *Aging Well*. New York: Little, Brown and Co.

Vaillant, G.E. (2008). *Spiritual Evolution: How We Are Wired for Faith, Hope, and Love*. New York: Broadway Books.

Van Deurzen, E. (1990) 'Existential therapy', in Dryden, W. (ed.) *Individual Therapy: A Handbook*. Milton Keynes, England: Open University Press, pp.149–174.

Van Deurzen, E. (1998) *Paradox and Passion in Psychotherapy*. Chichester: Wiley

Van Deurzen, E. (2010) *Everyday Mysteries: A Handbook of Existential Psychotherapy*. London & New York: Routledge.

Van Deurzen, E. (2012) *Existential Counselling and Psychotherapy in Practice* (3rd ed.). London: Sage.

Van Deurzen, E. & Adams, M. (2016) *Skills in Existential Counselling and Psychotherapy*. London: Sage.

Van Deurzen, E. & Arnold-Baker, C. (2018) *Existential Therapy: Distinctive Features*. London: Routledge.

Van Deurzen, E. & Iacovou, S. (2013) *Existential perspectives on relationship therapy*. Basingstoke: Palgrave Macmillan.

Van Deurzen, E. & Kenward, R. (2005) *Dictionary of Existential Counselling and Psychotherapy*. London: Sage.

Van Rijn, B. (2021a) 'Editor's Summary and reflection on sexual attraction and orientation in supervision', in Van Rijn, B. & Lukac-Greenwood, J. (eds) *Working with Sexual Attraction in Psychotherapy Practice and Supervision: A Humanistic-Relational Approach*. London: Routledge, pp.152–158.

Van Rijn, B. (2021b) 'Editor's Summary and reflection on ethical practice and prevention of transgressions', in Van Rijn, B. & Lukac-Greenwood, J. (eds) *Working with Sexual Attraction in Psychotherapy Practice and Supervision: A Humanistic-Relational Approach*. London: Routledge, pp.216–222.

Wahl, W. (2003) 'Working with "Existence Tension" as a Basis for Therapeutic Practice', *Existential Analysis Journal*, 14(2).

Welford, E. (2014) 'Giving the Dead Their Rightful Place', *Transactional Analysis Journal*, 44(4), pp.320–333. DOI:10.1177/0362153714559920

White, T. (1999) 'No-Psychosis Contracts', *Transactional Analysis Journal*, 29(2), pp.133–138. https://doi.org/10.1177/036215379902900207

White, T. (2001) 'The Contact Contract', *Transactional Analysis Journal*, *31*(3), pp.194–198. https://doi.org/10.1177/036215370103100308

White, T. (2022) 'Hard contracts, soft contracts and the unconscious', *International Journal of Transactional Analysis Research & Practice*, *13*(2), pp.25–31. https://doi.org/10.29044/v13i2p25

Widdowson, M (2008) 'Metacommunicative Transactions', *Transactional Analysis Journal*, 38(1), pp.58–71.

Wilde, O. (1891/1913). *The Picture of Dorian Gray*. London: Simpkin, Marshall, Hamilton, Kent and Company Limited.

Williams, P. (2002) *The Authority of Tenderness: Dignity and the True Self*. London & New York: Routledge.

Wink, P., & Dillon, M. (2002) 'Spiritual development across the adult life course: Findings from a longitudinal study', *Journal of Adult Development*, *9*(1), pp.79–94. https://doi.org/10.1023/A:1013833419122

Winnicott, D. W. (1958) 'The capacity to be alone', *The International Journal of Psychoanalysis*, *39*, pp.416–420.

Winnicott, D. W. (1960) 'The Theory of the Parent-Infant Relationship', *International Journal of Psychoanalysis 41*, pp.585–595.

Winnicott, D. W. (1963) 'Dependence in infant care, in child care, and in the psycho-analytic setting', *The International Journal of Psychoanalysis*, *44*(3), pp.339–344.

Winnicott, D. W. (1965) *The Maturational Processes and the Facilitating Environment: Studies in the Theory of Emotional Development*. Madison, Connecticut: International Universities Press.

Winnicott, D. W. (1989) *D. W. Winnicott: Psycho-analytic explorations* (eds. C. Winnicott, R. Shepard & M. Davis). Boston: Harvard University Press.

Wollheim, R. (1984) *The Thread of Life*. Cambridge, Massachusetts: Harvard University Press.

Wood, A. (2005) 'Alienation', in Honderich, T. (ed.) *The Oxford Companion to Philosophy*. Oxford: Oxford University Press.

Woods, H. (1926) *When the red, red robin (Comes bob, bob, bobbin' along)*. Brunswick Record Label.

Woods, K. (2005) 'The Therapist and the Erotic', *Transactional Analysis Journal*, *35*(3), pp.260–261. DOI:10.1177/036215370503500306

Woollams, S. & Brown, M. (1978) *Transactional Analysis*. Dexter, Michigan: Huron Valley Institute Press.

Woolf, V. (1927) *To the Lighthouse*. London: Hogarth Press.

Woolf, V. (1986) *The Essays of Virginia Woolf: 1912–1918*. London: Chatto & Windus.

Woolfe, R. & Biggs, S. (1997) 'Counselling older adults: issues and awareness', *Counselling Psychology Quarterly*, 10(2), pp.189–194.

Wordsworth, W. (1994) '"The Fountain: A Conversation", Poems of Sentiment and Reflection', in *The Collected Poems of William Wordsworth*. Hertfordshire, UK: Wordsworth Editions Ltd.

World Health Organization (2024) 'Ageing and Health'. Online factsheet. https://www.who.int/news-room/fact-sheets/detail/ageing-and-health

Yalom, I. (1980) *Existential Psychotherapy*. New York: Basic Books.

Yalom, I. D. (1985) *The theory and practice of group psychotherapy* (3rd ed.). Basic Books.

Yalom, I. D. (2002) *The Gift of Therapy: An Open Letter to a New Generation of Therapists and their Patients*. New York & London: HarperCollins Publishers.

Yalom, I. (2011) *Staring at the Sun: Being at Peace with Your Own Mortality: Overcoming the Terror of Death*. London: Piatkus.

Yetim, U. (2003) 'The impacts of individualism/collectivism, self-esteem, and feeling of mastery on life satisfaction among the Turkish university students and academicians', *Social Indicators Research*, *61*(3), pp.297–317. https://doi.org/10.1023/A:1021911504113

Index

Note: Locators in *italic* indicate figures and in ***bold-italic*** boxes.

For Product Safety Concerns and Information please contact our EU
representative GPSR@taylorandfrancis.com
Taylor & Francis Verlag GmbH, Kaufingerstraße 24, 80331 München, Germany

www.ingramcontent.com/pod-product-compliance
Lightning Source LLC
Chambersburg PA
CBHW070356270326
41926CB00014B/2578

9 781032 756912